Table of Contents

Mometrix
TEST PREPARATION

NBCE® Part I
Exam Secrets
Study Guide

Dear Future Exam Success Story

First of all, **THANK YOU** for purchasing Mometrix study materials!

Second, congratulations! You are one of the few determined test-takers who are committed to doing whatever it takes to excel on your exam. **You have come to the right place.** We developed these study materials with one goal in mind: to deliver you the information you need in a format that's concise and easy to use.

In addition to optimizing your guide for the content of the test, we've outlined our recommended steps for breaking down the preparation process into small, attainable goals so you can make sure you stay on track.

We've also analyzed the entire test-taking process, identifying the most common pitfalls and showing how you can overcome them and be ready for any curveball the test throws you.

Standardized testing is one of the biggest obstacles on your road to success, which only increases the importance of doing well in the high-pressure, high-stakes environment of test day. Your results on this test could have a significant impact on your future, and this guide provides the information and practical advice to help you achieve your full potential on test day.

Your success is our success

We would love to hear from you! If you would like to share the story of your exam success or if you have any questions or comments in regard to our products, please contact us at **800-673-8175** or **support@mometrix.com**.

Thanks again for your business and we wish you continued success!

Sincerely,
The Mometrix Test Preparation Team

Need more help? Check out our flashcards at:
http://MometrixFlashcards.com/NBCE

Written and edited by the Mometrix Exam Secrets Test Prep Team
Printed in the United States of America

Introduction

Thank you for purchasing this resource! You have made the choice to prepare yourself for a test that could have a huge impact on your future, and this guide is designed to help you be fully ready for test day. Obviously, it's important to have a solid understanding of the test material, but you also need to be prepared for the unique environment and stressors of the test, so that you can perform to the best of your abilities.

For this purpose, the first section that appears in this guide is the **Secret Keys**. We've devoted countless hours to meticulously researching what works and what doesn't, and we've boiled down our findings to the five most impactful steps you can take to improve your performance on the test. We start at the beginning with study planning and move through the preparation process, all the way to the testing strategies that will help you get the most out of what you know when you're finally sitting in front of the test.

We recommend that you start preparing for your test as far in advance as possible. However, if you've bought this guide as a last-minute study resource and only have a few days before your test, we recommend that you skip over the first two Secret Keys since they address a long-term study plan.

If you struggle with **test anxiety**, we strongly encourage you to check out our recommendations for how you can overcome it. Test anxiety is a formidable foe, but it can be beaten, and we want to make sure you have the tools you need to defeat it.

Secret Key #1 – Plan Big, Study Small

There's a lot riding on your performance. If you want to ace this test, you're going to need to keep your skills sharp and the material fresh in your mind. You need a plan that lets you review everything you need to know while still fitting in your schedule. We'll break this strategy down into three categories.

Information Organization

Start with the information you already have: the official test outline. From this, you can make a complete list of all the concepts you need to cover before the test. Organize these concepts into groups that can be studied together, and create a list of any related vocabulary you need to learn so you can brush up on any difficult terms. You'll want to keep this vocabulary list handy once you actually start studying since you may need to add to it along the way.

Time Management

Once you have your set of study concepts, decide how to spread them out over the time you have left before the test. Break your study plan into small, clear goals so you have a manageable task for each day and know exactly what you're doing. Then just focus on one small step at a time. When you manage your time this way, you don't need to spend hours at a time studying. Studying a small block of content for a short period each day helps you retain information better and avoid stressing over how much you have left to do. You can relax knowing that you have a plan to cover everything in time. In order for this strategy to be effective though, you have to start studying early and stick to your schedule. Avoid the exhaustion and futility that comes from last-minute cramming!

Study Environment

The environment you study in has a big impact on your learning. Studying in a coffee shop, while probably more enjoyable, is not likely to be as fruitful as studying in a quiet room. It's important to keep distractions to a minimum. You're only planning to study for a short block of time, so make the most of it. Don't pause to check your phone or get up to find a snack. It's also important to **avoid multitasking**. Research has consistently shown that multitasking will make your studying dramatically less effective. Your study area should also be comfortable and well-lit so you don't have the distraction of straining your eyes or sitting on an uncomfortable chair.

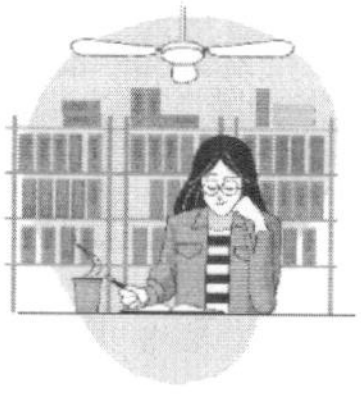

The time of day you study is also important. You want to be rested and alert. Don't wait until just before bedtime. Study when you'll be most likely to comprehend and remember. Even better, if you know what time of day your test will be, set that time aside for study. That way your brain will be used to working on that subject at that specific time and you'll have a better chance of recalling information.

Finally, it can be helpful to team up with others who are studying for the same test. Your actual studying should be done in as isolated an environment as possible, but the work of organizing the information and setting up the study plan can be divided up. In between study sessions, you can discuss with your teammates the concepts that you're all studying and quiz each other on the details. Just be sure that your teammates are as serious about the test as you are. If you find that your study time is being replaced with social time, you might need to find a new team.

Secret Key #2 – Make Your Studying Count

You're devoting a lot of time and effort to preparing for this test, so you want to be absolutely certain it will pay off. This means doing more than just reading the content and hoping you can remember it on test day. It's important to make every minute of study count. There are two main areas you can focus on to make your studying count.

Retention

It doesn't matter how much time you study if you can't remember the material. You need to make sure you are retaining the concepts. To check your retention of the information you're learning, try recalling it at later times with minimal prompting. Try carrying around flashcards and glance at one or two from time to time or ask a friend who's also studying for the test to quiz you.

To enhance your retention, look for ways to put the information into practice so that you can apply it rather than simply recalling it. If you're using the information in practical ways, it will be much easier to remember. Similarly, it helps to solidify a concept in your mind if you're not only reading it to yourself but also explaining it to someone else. Ask a friend to let you teach them about a concept you're a little shaky on (or speak aloud to an imaginary audience if necessary). As you try to summarize, define, give examples, and answer your friend's questions, you'll understand the concepts better and they will stay with you longer. Finally, step back for a big picture view and ask yourself how each piece of information fits with the whole subject. When you link the different concepts together and see them working together as a whole, it's easier to remember the individual components.

Finally, practice showing your work on any multi-step problems, even if you're just studying. Writing out each step you take to solve a problem will help solidify the process in your mind, and you'll be more likely to remember it during the test.

Modality

Modality simply refers to the means or method by which you study. Choosing a study modality that fits your own individual learning style is crucial. No two people learn best in exactly the same way, so it's important to know your strengths and use them to your advantage.

For example, if you learn best by visualization, focus on visualizing a concept in your mind and draw an image or a diagram. Try color-coding your notes, illustrating them, or creating symbols that will trigger your mind to recall a learned concept. If you learn best by hearing or discussing information, find a study partner who learns the same way or read aloud to yourself. Think about how to put the information in your own words. Imagine that you are giving a lecture on the topic and record yourself so you can listen to it later.

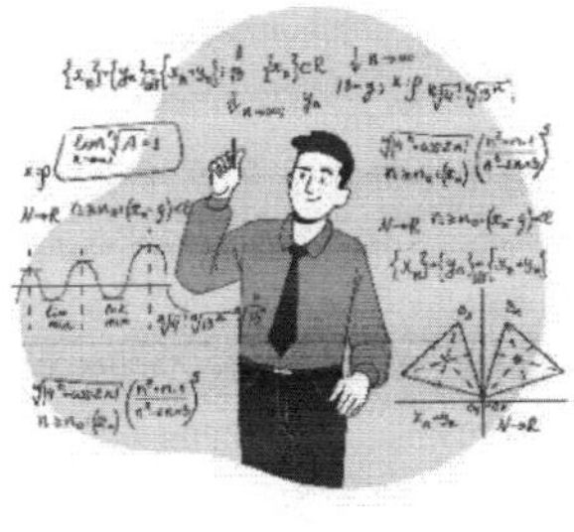

For any learning style, flashcards can be helpful. Organize the information so you can take advantage of spare moments to review. Underline key words or phrases. Use different colors for different categories. Mnemonic devices (such as creating a short list in which every item starts with the same letter) can also help with retention. Find what works best for you and use it to store the information in your mind most effectively and easily.

Secret Key #3 – Practice the Right Way

Your success on test day depends not only on how many hours you put into preparing, but also on whether you prepared the right way. It's good to check along the way to see if your studying is paying off. One of the most effective ways to do this is by taking practice tests to evaluate your progress. Practice tests are useful because they show exactly where you need to improve. Every time you take a practice test, pay special attention to these three groups of questions:

- The questions you got wrong
- The questions you had to guess on, even if you guessed right
- The questions you found difficult or slow to work through

This will show you exactly what your weak areas are, and where you need to devote more study time. Ask yourself why each of these questions gave you trouble. Was it because you didn't understand the material? Was it because you didn't remember the vocabulary? Do you need more repetitions on this type of question to build speed and confidence? Dig into those questions and figure out how you can strengthen your weak areas as you go back to review the material.

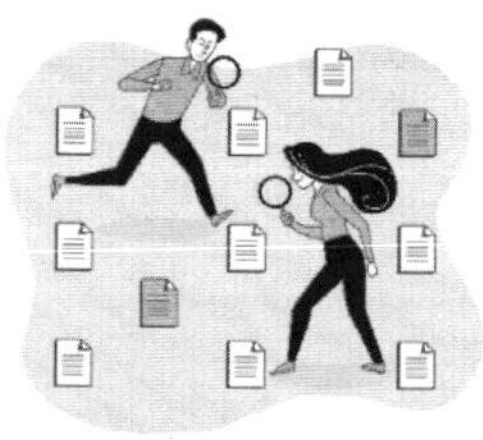

Additionally, many practice tests have a section explaining the answer choices. It can be tempting to read the explanation and think that you now have a good understanding of the concept. However, an explanation likely only covers part of the question's broader context. Even if the explanation makes perfect sense, **go back and investigate** every concept related to the question until you're positive you have a thorough understanding.

As you go along, keep in mind that the practice test is just that: practice. Memorizing these questions and answers will not be very helpful on the actual test because it is unlikely to have any of the same exact questions. If you only know the right answers to the sample questions, you won't be prepared for the real thing. **Study the concepts** until you understand them fully, and then you'll be able to answer any question that shows up on the test.

It's important to wait on the practice tests until you're ready. If you take a test on your first day of study, you may be overwhelmed by the amount of material covered and how much you need to learn. Work up to it gradually.

On test day, you'll need to be prepared for answering questions, managing your time, and using the test-taking strategies you've learned. It's a lot to balance, like a mental marathon that will have a big impact on your future. Like training for a marathon, you'll need to start slowly and work your way up. When test day arrives, you'll be ready.

Start with the strategies you've read in the first two Secret Keys—plan your course and study in the way that works best for you. If you have time, consider using multiple study resources to get different approaches to the same concepts. It can be helpful to see difficult concepts from more than one angle. Then find a good source for practice tests. Many times, the test website will suggest potential study resources or provide sample tests.

Practice Test Strategy

If you're able to find at least three practice tests, we recommend this strategy:

Untimed and Open-Book Practice

Take the first test with no time constraints and with your notes and study guide handy. Take your time and focus on applying the strategies you've learned.

Timed and Open-Book Practice

Take the second practice test open-book as well, but set a timer and practice pacing yourself to finish in time.

Timed and Closed-Book Practice

Take any other practice tests as if it were test day. Set a timer and put away your study materials. Sit at a table or desk in a quiet room, imagine yourself at the testing center, and answer questions as quickly and accurately as possible.

Keep repeating timed and closed-book tests on a regular basis until you run out of practice tests or it's time for the actual test. Your mind will be ready for the schedule and stress of test day, and you'll be able to focus on recalling the material you've learned.

Secret Key #4 – Pace Yourself

Once you're fully prepared for the material on the test, your biggest challenge on test day will be managing your time. Just knowing that the clock is ticking can make you panic even if you have plenty of time left. Work on pacing yourself so you can build confidence against the time constraints of the exam. Pacing is a difficult skill to master, especially in a high-pressure environment, so **practice is vital**.

Set time expectations for your pace based on how much time is available. For example, if a section has 60 questions and the time limit is 30 minutes, you know you have to average 30 seconds or less per question in order to answer them all. Although 30 seconds is the hard limit, set 25 seconds per question as your goal, so you reserve extra time to spend on harder questions. When you budget extra time for the harder questions, you no longer have any reason to stress when those questions take longer to answer.

Don't let this time expectation distract you from working through the test at a calm, steady pace, but keep it in mind so you don't spend too much time on any one question. Recognize that taking extra time on one question you don't understand may keep you from answering two that you do understand later in the test. If your time limit for a question is up and you're still not sure of the answer, mark it and move on, and come back to it later if the time and the test format allow. If the testing format doesn't allow you to return to earlier questions, just make an educated guess; then put it out of your mind and move on.

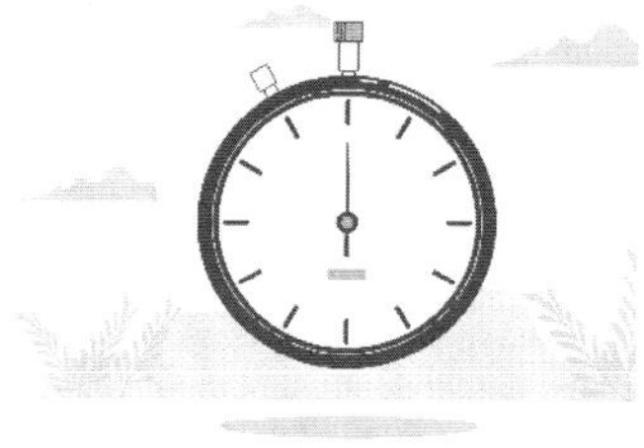

On the easier questions, be careful not to rush. It may seem wise to hurry through them so you have more time for the challenging ones, but it's not worth missing one if you know the concept and just didn't take the time to read the question fully. Work efficiently but make sure you understand the question and have looked at all of the answer choices, since more than one may seem right at first.

Even if you're paying attention to the time, you may find yourself a little behind at some point. You should speed up to get back on track, but do so wisely. Don't panic; just take a few seconds less on each question until you're caught up. Don't guess without thinking, but do look through the answer choices and eliminate any you know are wrong. If you can get down to two choices, it is often worthwhile to guess from those. Once you've chosen an answer, move on and don't dwell on any that you skipped or had to hurry through. If a question was taking too long, chances are it was one of the harder ones, so you weren't as likely to get it right anyway.

On the other hand, if you find yourself getting ahead of schedule, it may be beneficial to slow down a little. The more quickly you work, the more likely you are to make a careless mistake that will affect your score. You've budgeted time for each question, so don't be afraid to spend that time. Practice an efficient but careful pace to get the most out of the time you have.

Secret Key #5 – Have a Plan for Guessing

When you're taking the test, you may find yourself stuck on a question. Some of the answer choices seem better than others, but you don't see the one answer choice that is obviously correct. What do you do?

The scenario described above is very common, yet most test takers have not effectively prepared for it. Developing and practicing a plan for guessing may be one of the single most effective uses of your time as you get ready for the exam.

In developing your plan for guessing, there are three questions to address:

- When should you start the guessing process?
- How should you narrow down the choices?
- Which answer should you choose?

When to Start the Guessing Process

Unless your plan for guessing is to select C every time (which, despite its merits, is not what we recommend), you need to leave yourself enough time to apply your answer elimination strategies. Since you have a limited amount of time for each question, that means that if you're going to give yourself the best shot at guessing correctly, you have to decide quickly whether or not you will guess.

Of course, the best-case scenario is that you don't have to guess at all, so first, see if you can answer the question based on your knowledge of the subject and basic reasoning skills. Focus on the key words in the question and try to jog your memory of related topics. Give yourself a chance to bring the knowledge to mind, but once you realize that you don't have (or you can't access) the knowledge you need to answer the question, it's time to start the guessing process.

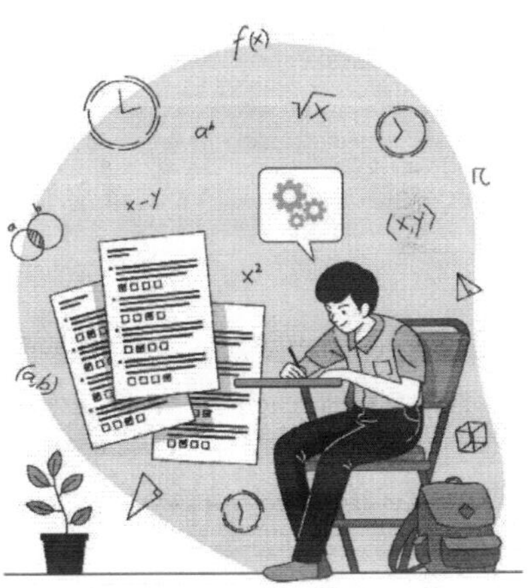

It's almost always better to start the guessing process too early than too late. It only takes a few seconds to remember something and answer the question from knowledge. Carefully eliminating wrong answer choices takes longer. Plus, going through the process of eliminating answer choices can actually help jog your memory.

Summary: Start the guessing process as soon as you decide that you can't answer the question based on your knowledge.

How to Narrow Down the Choices

The next chapter in this book (**Test-Taking Strategies**) includes a wide range of strategies for how to approach questions and how to look for answer choices to eliminate. You will definitely want to read those carefully, practice them, and figure out which ones work best for you. Here though, we're going to address a mindset rather than a particular strategy.

Your odds of guessing an answer correctly depend on how many options you are choosing from.

Number of options left	5	4	3	2	1
Odds of guessing correctly	20%	25%	33%	50%	100%

You can see from this chart just how valuable it is to be able to eliminate incorrect answers and make an educated guess, but there are two things that many test takers do that cause them to miss out on the benefits of guessing:

- Accidentally eliminating the correct answer
- Selecting an answer based on an impression

We'll look at the first one here, and the second one in the next section.

To avoid accidentally eliminating the correct answer, we recommend a thought exercise called **the $5 challenge**. In this challenge, you only eliminate an answer choice from contention if you are willing to bet $5 on it being wrong. Why $5? Five dollars is a small but not insignificant amount of money. It's an amount you could afford to lose but wouldn't want to throw away. And while losing $5 once might not hurt too much, doing it twenty times will set you back $100. In the same way, each small decision you make—eliminating a choice here, guessing on a question there—won't by itself impact your score very much, but when you put them all together, they can make a big difference. By holding each answer choice elimination decision to a higher standard, you can reduce the risk of accidentally eliminating the correct answer.

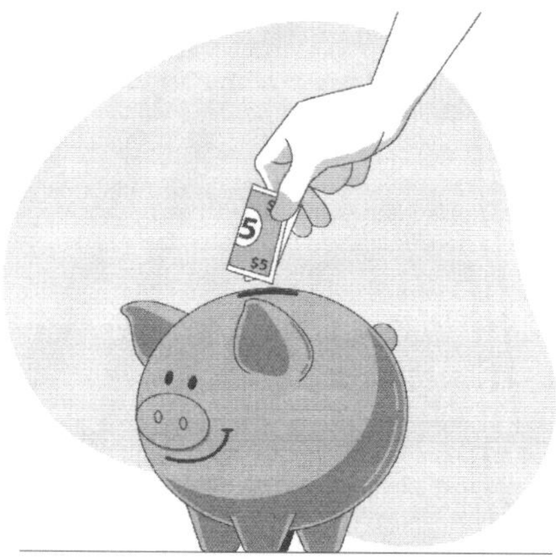

The $5 challenge can also be applied in a positive sense: If you are willing to bet $5 that an answer choice *is* correct, go ahead and mark it as correct.

Summary: Only eliminate an answer choice if you are willing to bet $5 that it is wrong.

Which Answer to Choose

You're taking the test. You've run into a hard question and decided you'll have to guess. You've eliminated all the answer choices you're willing to bet $5 on. Now you have to pick an answer. Why do we even need to talk about this? Why can't you just pick whichever one you feel like when the time comes?

The answer to these questions is that if you don't come into the test with a plan, you'll rely on your impression to select an answer choice, and if you do that, you risk falling into a trap. The test writers know that everyone who takes their test will be guessing on some of the questions, so they intentionally write wrong answer choices to seem plausible. You still have to pick an answer though, and if the wrong answer choices are designed to look right, how can you ever be sure that you're not falling for their trap? The best solution we've found to this dilemma is to take the decision out of your hands entirely. Here is the process we recommend:

Once you've eliminated any choices that you are confident (willing to bet $5) are wrong, select the first remaining choice as your answer.

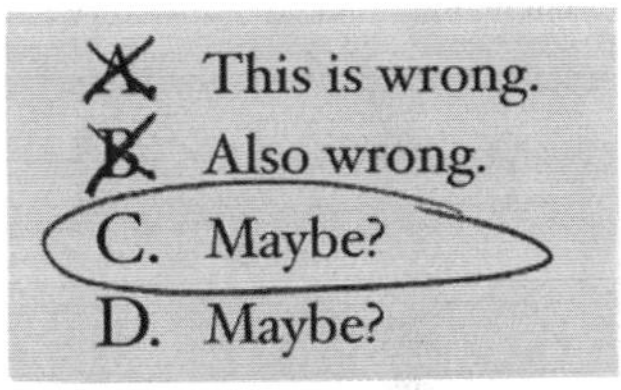

Whether you choose to select the first remaining choice, the second, or the last, the important thing is that you use some preselected standard. Using this approach guarantees that you will not be enticed into selecting an answer choice that looks right, because you are not basing your decision on how the answer choices look.

This is not meant to make you question your knowledge. Instead, it is to help you recognize the difference between your knowledge and your impressions. There's a huge difference between thinking an answer is right because of what you know, and thinking an answer is right because it looks or sounds like it should be right.

Summary: To ensure that your selection is appropriately random, make a predetermined selection from among all answer choices you have not eliminated.

Test-Taking Strategies

This section contains a list of test-taking strategies that you may find helpful as you work through the test. By taking what you know and applying logical thought, you can maximize your chances of answering any question correctly!

It is very important to realize that every question is different and every person is different: no single strategy will work on every question, and no single strategy will work for every person. That's why we've included all of them here, so you can try them out and determine which ones work best for different types of questions and which ones work best for you.

Question Strategies

✓ Read Carefully

Read the question and the answer choices carefully. Don't miss the question because you misread the terms. You have plenty of time to read each question thoroughly and make sure you understand what is being asked. Yet a happy medium must be attained, so don't waste too much time. You must read carefully and efficiently.

✓ Contextual Clues

Look for contextual clues. If the question includes a word you are not familiar with, look at the immediate context for some indication of what the word might mean. Contextual clues can often give you all the information you need to decipher the meaning of an unfamiliar word. Even if you can't determine the meaning, you may be able to narrow down the possibilities enough to make a solid guess at the answer to the question.

✓ Prefixes

If you're having trouble with a word in the question or answer choices, try dissecting it. Take advantage of every clue that the word might include. Prefixes can be a huge help. Usually, they allow you to determine a basic meaning. *Pre-* means before, *post-* means after, *pro-* is positive, *de-* is negative. From prefixes, you can get an idea of the general meaning of the word and try to put it into context.

✓ Hedge Words

Watch out for critical hedge words, such as *likely, may, can, often, almost, mostly, usually, generally, rarely,* and *sometimes.* Question writers insert these hedge phrases to cover every possibility. Often an answer choice will be wrong simply because it leaves no room for exception. Be on guard for answer choices that have definitive words such as *exactly* and *always.*

✓ Switchback Words

Stay alert for *switchbacks.* These are the words and phrases frequently used to alert you to shifts in thought. The most common switchback words are *but, although,* and *however.* Others include *nevertheless, on the other hand, even though, while, in spite of, despite,* and *regardless of.* Switchback words are important to catch because they can change the direction of the question or an answer choice.

☑ Face Value

When in doubt, use common sense. Accept the situation in the problem at face value. Don't read too much into it. These problems will not require you to make wild assumptions. If you have to go beyond creativity and warp time or space in order to have an answer choice fit the question, then you should move on and consider the other answer choices. These are normal problems rooted in reality. The applicable relationship or explanation may not be readily apparent, but it is there for you to figure out. Use your common sense to interpret anything that isn't clear.

Answer Choice Strategies

☑ Answer Selection

The most thorough way to pick an answer choice is to identify and eliminate wrong answers until only one is left, then confirm it is the correct answer. Sometimes an answer choice may immediately seem right, but be careful. The test writers will usually put more than one reasonable answer choice on each question, so take a second to read all of them and make sure that the other choices are not equally obvious. As long as you have time left, it is better to read every answer choice than to pick the first one that looks right without checking the others.

☑ Answer Choice Families

An answer choice family consists of two (in rare cases, three) answer choices that are very similar in construction and cannot all be true at the same time. If you see two answer choices that are direct opposites or parallels, one of them is usually the correct answer. For instance, if one answer choice says that quantity x increases and another either says that quantity x decreases (opposite) or says that quantity y increases (parallel), then those answer choices would fall into the same family. An answer choice that doesn't match the construction of the answer choice family is more likely to be incorrect. Most questions will not have answer choice families, but when they do appear, you should be prepared to recognize them.

☑ Eliminate Answers

Eliminate answer choices as soon as you realize they are wrong, but make sure you consider all possibilities. If you are eliminating answer choices and realize that the last one you are left with is also wrong, don't panic. Start over and consider each choice again. There may be something you missed the first time that you will realize on the second pass.

☑ Avoid Fact Traps

Don't be distracted by an answer choice that is factually true but doesn't answer the question. You are looking for the choice that answers the question. Stay focused on what the question is asking for so you don't accidentally pick an answer that is true but incorrect. Always go back to the question and make sure the answer choice you've selected actually answers the question and is not merely a true statement.

☑ Extreme Statements

In general, you should avoid answers that put forth extreme actions as standard practice or proclaim controversial ideas as established fact. An answer choice that states the "process should be used in certain situations, if…" is much more likely to be correct than one that states the "process should be discontinued completely." The first is a calm rational statement and doesn't even make a definitive, uncompromising stance, using a hedge word *if* to provide wiggle room, whereas the second choice is far more extreme.

⊘ Benchmark

As you read through the answer choices and you come across one that seems to answer the question well, mentally select that answer choice. This is not your final answer, but it's the one that will help you evaluate the other answer choices. The one that you selected is your benchmark or standard for judging each of the other answer choices. Every other answer choice must be compared to your benchmark. That choice is correct until proven otherwise by another answer choice beating it. If you find a better answer, then that one becomes your new benchmark. Once you've decided that no other choice answers the question as well as your benchmark, you have your final answer.

⊘ Predict the Answer

Before you even start looking at the answer choices, it is often best to try to predict the answer. When you come up with the answer on your own, it is easier to avoid distractions and traps because you will know exactly what to look for. The right answer choice is unlikely to be word-for-word what you came up with, but it should be a close match. Even if you are confident that you have the right answer, you should still take the time to read each option before moving on.

General Strategies

⊘ Tough Questions

If you are stumped on a problem or it appears too hard or too difficult, don't waste time. Move on! Remember though, if you can quickly check for obviously incorrect answer choices, your chances of guessing correctly are greatly improved. Before you completely give up, at least try to knock out a couple of possible answers. Eliminate what you can and then guess at the remaining answer choices before moving on.

⊘ Check Your Work

Since you will probably not know every term listed and the answer to every question, it is important that you get credit for the ones that you do know. Don't miss any questions through careless mistakes. If at all possible, try to take a second to look back over your answer selection and make sure you've selected the correct answer choice and haven't made a costly careless mistake (such as marking an answer choice that you didn't mean to mark). This quick double check should more than pay for itself in caught mistakes for the time it costs.

⊘ Pace Yourself

It's easy to be overwhelmed when you're looking at a page full of questions; your mind is confused and full of random thoughts, and the clock is ticking down faster than you would like. Calm down and maintain the pace that you have set for yourself. Especially as you get down to the last few minutes of the test, don't let the small numbers on the clock make you panic. As long as you are on track by monitoring your pace, you are guaranteed to have time for each question.

⊘ Don't Rush

It is very easy to make errors when you are in a hurry. Maintaining a fast pace in answering questions is pointless if it makes you miss questions that you would have gotten right otherwise. Test writers like to include distracting information and wrong answers that seem right. Taking a little extra time to avoid careless mistakes can make all the difference in your test score. Find a pace that allows you to be confident in the answers that you select.

⊘ KEEP MOVING

Panicking will not help you pass the test, so do your best to stay calm and keep moving. Taking deep breaths and going through the answer elimination steps you practiced can help to break through a stress barrier and keep your pace.

Final Notes

The combination of a solid foundation of content knowledge and the confidence that comes from practicing your plan for applying that knowledge is the key to maximizing your performance on test day. As your foundation of content knowledge is built up and strengthened, you'll find that the strategies included in this chapter become more and more effective in helping you quickly sift through the distractions and traps of the test to isolate the correct answer.

Now that you're preparing to move forward into the test content chapters of this book, be sure to keep your goal in mind. As you read, think about how you will be able to apply this information on the test. If you've already seen sample questions for the test and you have an idea of the question format and style, try to come up with questions of your own that you can answer based on what you're reading. This will give you valuable practice applying your knowledge in the same ways you can expect to on test day.

Good luck and good studying!

General Anatomy

Anatomical Planes of the Human Body

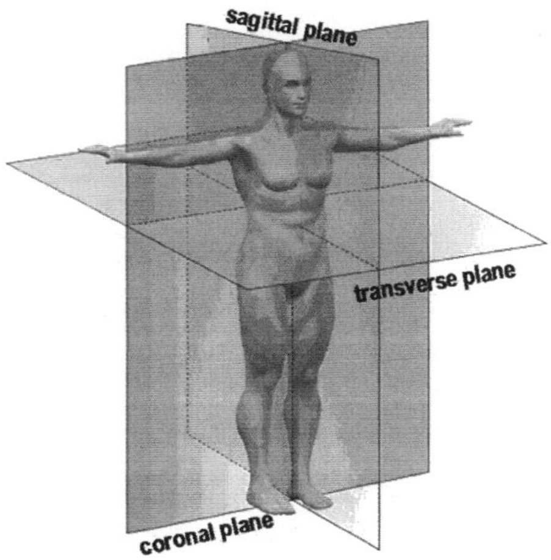

Muscles of the Head and Neck

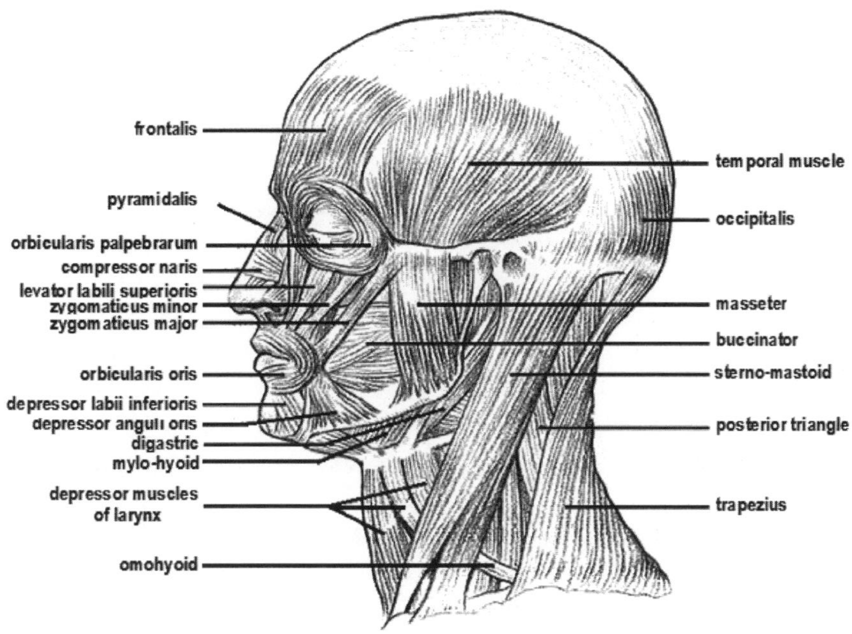

Perineum

The perineum—the pelvic outlet—is the area between the legs at the base of the trunk and the structures associated with this area. It is found in both sexes. In a transverse plane view, it is bordered anteriorly by the pubic symphysis, laterally by the ischial tuberosities, and posteriorly by the coccyx. In a superficial view, it is the region lying between the posterior margins of the genitalia (the scrotum in males and the posterior junction of the vulva in females) and the anus.

Superficial perineum in females:

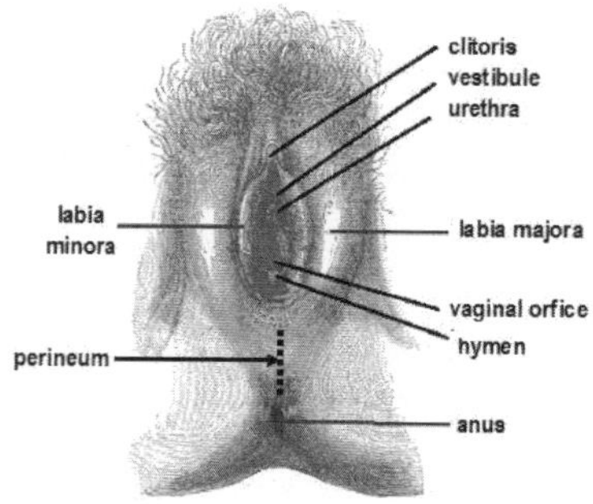

Human Pelvis

The pelvis is a basin-shaped structure formed by the two lateroventral innominate bones (each consisting of an anterior pubis and an ilium, as well as an ischium), the posterior sacrum, and the coccyx. In males, the pelvis is heart-shaped, and is larger and heavier than the female pelvis. The female pelvis is relatively smaller, but is wider and rounder to facilitate childbirth. There is a great deal of variation among individuals, however.

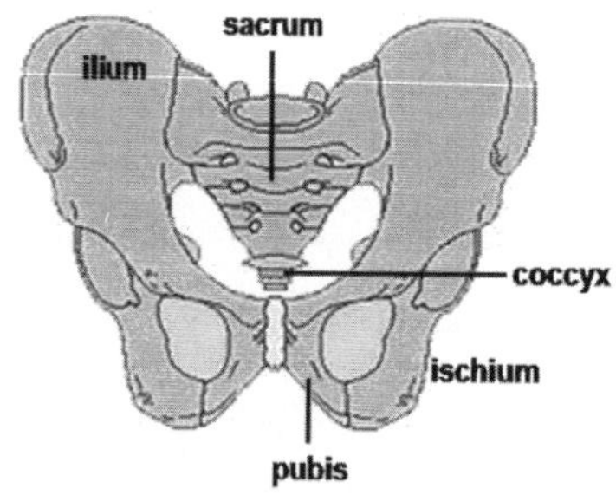

Axial Skeleton and Appendicular Skeleton

The axial skeleton (shown in black in the figure) consists of the skull, the spinal column, and the ribcage. The appendicular skeleton (shown in grey) consists of the pectoral or shoulder girdle (the scapula and the clavicle) and the pelvic girdle (the fused innominate bone plus the sacrum and attached coccyx), as well as the upper and lower limb bones attached to the two girdles. The upper limb bones include the humerus, the radius, the ulna, and the bones of the wrist and hand. The lower limb bones include the femur, the tibia, the fibula, and the bones of the ankle and foot.

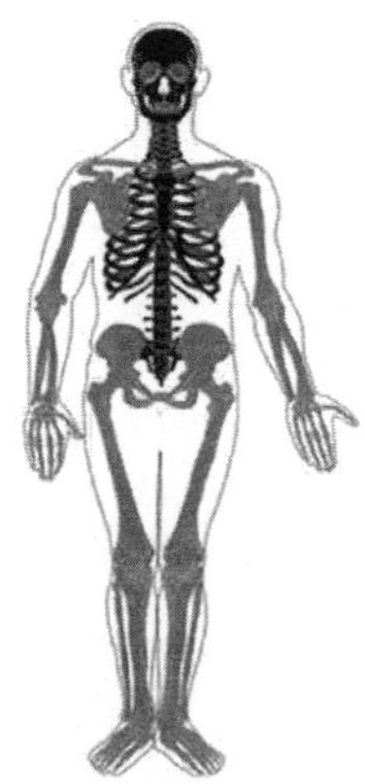

INTEGUMENTARY SYSTEM

The integument consists of the skin and its associated structures, such as hair, nails, and sweat glands. It is the largest organ in the body, covering an area of between one and a half and two square meters. It is comprised of three main layers: an outer epidermis derived from embryonic ectoderm and two underlying mesodermal layers. The middle layer is called the dermis, and the one below that is called the hypodermis. The epidermis is the outermost barrier between the organism and the environment. It consists mostly of dead or dying keratinized cells. It lacks blood vessels, and it obtains its nutrients and meets other requirements through diffusion of materials originating in the dermis. The dermis contains connective tissue and collagen, capillaries, muscles, nerve endings, sebaceous glands, and sweat gland ducts. The hypodermis consists mainly of adipose tissue. The sweat glands themselves are located at the boundary between the dermis and the hypodermis.

Review Video: Integumentary System
Visit mometrix.com/academy and enter code: 655980

LAYERS

Three main layers of the integument:

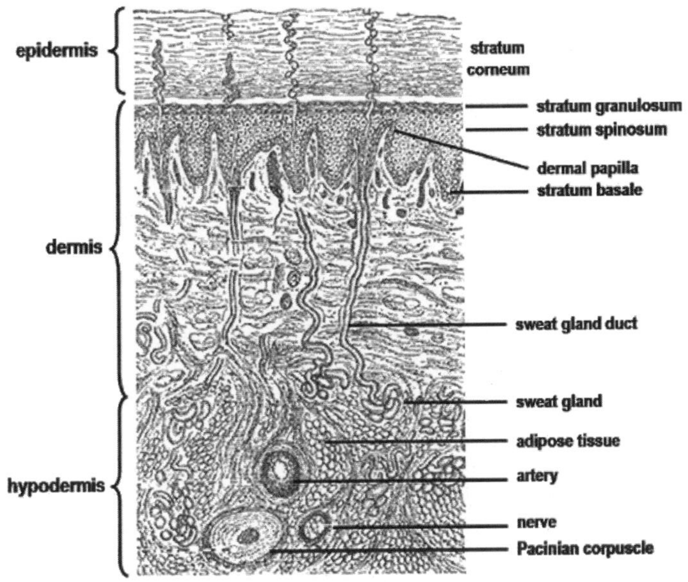

Epidermal Layers

Epidermal layers of the integument:

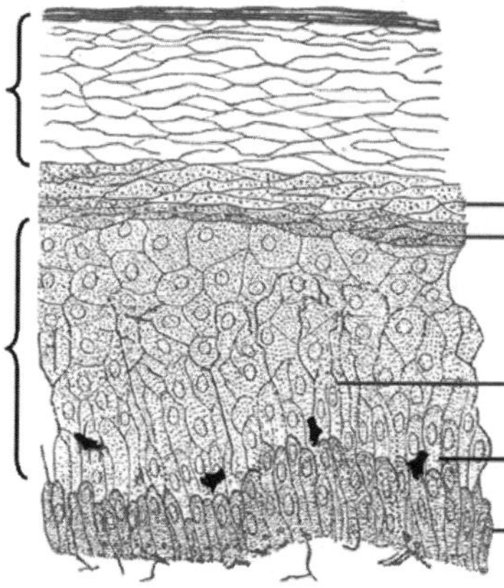

Compact Bone

The cylindrical osteon is the structural and functional unit of compact (cortical) bone. Each osteon consists of concentric layers (lamellae) of compact bone surrounding a central Haversian canal that contains blood vessels. Each osteon is about 0.2 mm in diameter. Small spaces called lacunae contain osteocytes (bone cells) connected by cytoplasmic extensions through tiny passageways called canaliculi. The osteons undergo constant remodeling as calcium is broken down and mobilized for use by the body, and later redeposited when it is no longer needed.

Osteon

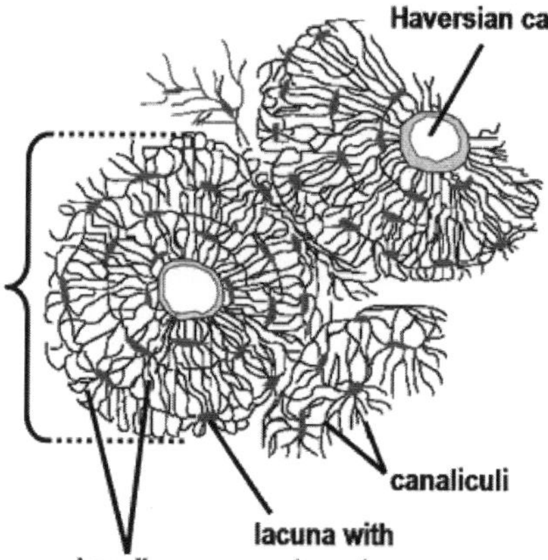

Spongy or Cancellous Bone

Spongy, cancellous, or trabecular bone is softer and much less dense than compact bone. It is highly vascularized, and contains red marrow where hematopoiesis (the formation of red blood cells) occurs. It consists of open spaces and connecting ridges and shelves called trabeculae. It is found at the ends of long bones and in the interiors of flat bones and vertebrae. It is the slight compressibility of spongy bone that allows the long bones of the body to bear the body's weight.

Relationships Between Compact and Spongy Bone

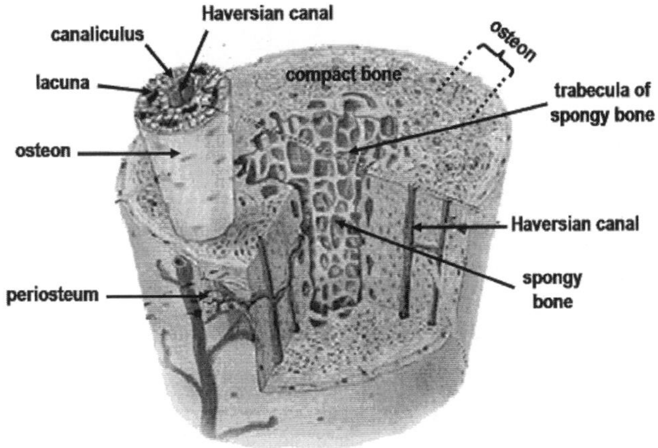

Dermal Bone and Endochondral Bone

Dermal bone (membrane bone) arises directly from the dermis, and is not preformed in cartilage. It forms the major part of the braincase and certain other structures on the skull, elements of the upper jaw (the premaxilla, maxilla, palatine, vomer, and pterygoid lamina), and the mandible (lower jaw). In humans, it also forms the clavicle (collarbone). Endochondral bone is preformed in cartilage, and is gradually replaced during prenatal and postnatal development by bone. Except for the clavicles, the entire skeleton below the skull is formed from endochondral bone.

Long Bones

Long bones are preformed by cartilage laid down by chondrocytes. The fibrous perichondrium surrounding the cartilage becomes the periosteum, which encloses all bones except the ends of the long bones. It produces osteoprogenitor cells that transform into osteoblasts, which begin laying down bone in the primary ossification center in the middle of the long bone's diaphysis (shaft). A cavity created in the primary ossification center by disintegrating chondrocytes is invaded by blood vessels from the periosteum. These blood vessels branch in both directions along the length of the diaphysis. They carry osteoprogenitor cells and hemopoietic cells into the growing cavity, which will later accumulate bone marrow. Secondary ossification centers appear at both ends (epiphyses) of the developing long bone. The epiphyses are separated from the diaphysis by a cartilaginous epiphyseal plate, which forms new cartilage that is replaced by bone as the long bone lengthens. When increases in body height cease at maturity, the epiphyseal plates become ossified into the epiphyseal line.

Features of a long bone:

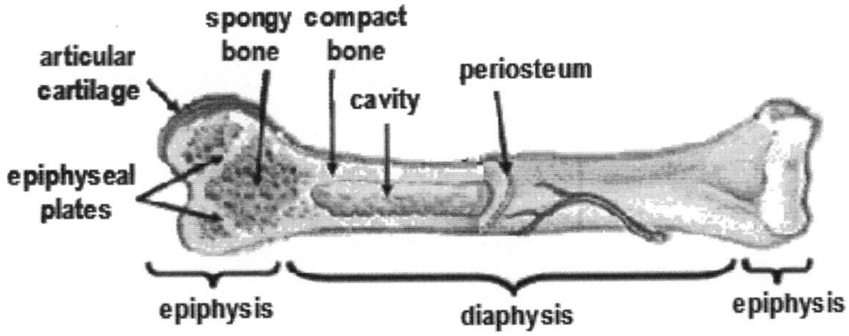

Human Pectoral Girdle

The pectoral (shoulder) girdle consists of the scapula (shoulder blade) and the clavicle (collar bone). The glenoid fossa of the scapula is connected with the head of the humerus by a synovial ball-and-socket joint called the glenohumeral joint. The pectoral girdle is attached to the sternum by the sternoclavicular joint; no joint exists between the scapula and the rib cage. These loose attachments allow for maximum mobility.

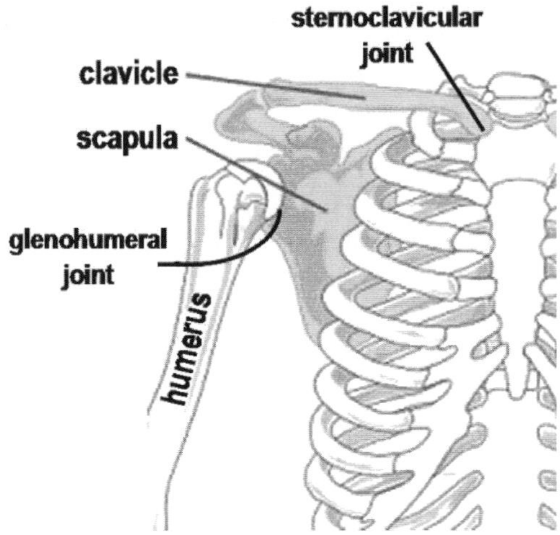

Human Pelvic Girdle

The *os coxa* refers to both the entire pelvis and the hip joint. The pelvis includes the two innominate bones (*ossa coxae*), each of which consist of the fused ilium, ischium, and pubis. They meet in and around the acetabulum. They are connected posteriorly by the sacrum and the coccyx, and anteriorly by the pubic symphysis. Each innominate bone has one of the few true ball-and-socket joints of the body: the cuplike acetabulum into which the head of the femur fits to form the acetabulofemoral joint. Both the femoral head and the acetabulum are covered by lubricated hyaline cartilage. In elderly persons suffering from osteoporosis, the neck connecting the femoral head to the femoral shaft is susceptible to subcapital fracture.

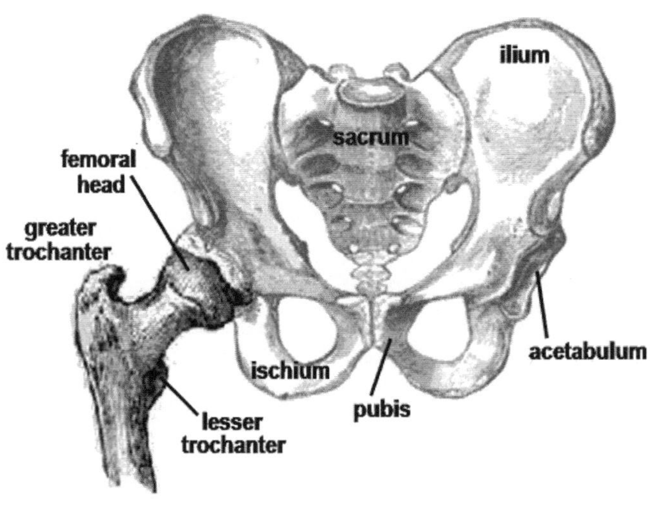

Os Coxa

Each *os coxa* of the adult pelvic girdle forms through the fusion of the ilium, the ischium, and the pubis, large portions of which are cartilage at birth. By age seven or eight, the inferior portions of the ischium and the pubis have become fused bone. Ossification of the remaining cartilage is complete by puberty, and the final fusion of all three elements occurs between ages 20 and 25. Bone density increases throughout childhood and adolescence, and bone mass peaks at age 25. It remains stable until middle age, at which time it begins to decline. For many, especially postmenopausal women, this can lead to osteopenia and then osteoporosis. A person who has osteoporosis will be at an increased risk of fractures for the rest of his or her life.

Bone Remodeling

Bone remodeling occurs throughout life. It promotes continued bone health and strength, and also allows for the repair of fractures. Old bone is continually resorbed and new bone laid down in its place, which results in a dynamic equilibrium. Imbalances between these two processes can result in a variety of bone disorders, such as osteoporosis, in later years. Osteoclasts and osteoblasts, both of which are derived from hematopoietic stem cells, dissolve old bone and lay down new bone, respectively. The complex signaling pathways that coordinate these two actions involve parathyroid hormone (PTH) from the parathyroid glands, a growth hormone, interleukin-6 (IL-6), steroid hormones, vitamin D3, and calcitonin from the thyroid gland. PTH increases the plasma concentration of Ca^{2+} by dissolving it from bone; calcitonin decreases it and lays it down into new bone. PTH stimulates both osteoclasts and osteoblasts, which interact via negative feedback pathways to destroy and lay down bone.

Joints

The categories of joints based on biomechanical function are as follows:

- Hinge joint — the simplest type of joint; allows movement in only one direction; an example is the elbow joint
- Pivot joint — allows for rotary motion; an example is the joint between the atlas and the axis
- Condylar joint — a joint with an ovoid surface within an elliptical cavity; the metacarpophalangeal joints are an example
- Gliding joints — similar to a swivel; allow for a wide range of movement; the vertebrae are an example
- Saddle joint — allows movement in two directions; the base of the thumb is an example
- Ball-and-socket joint — provides the greatest range of movement; the spherical head of one bone lies within the cuplike cavity of another; an example is the acetabulofemoral joint

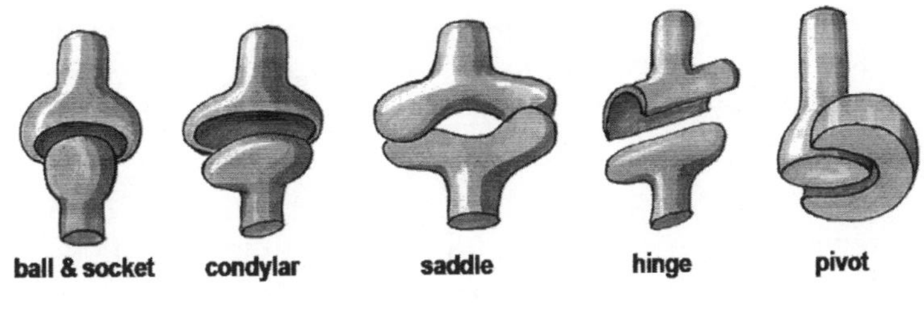

Levers

First-, second-, and third-class levers in the human body are as follows:

- First-class lever — The fulcrum lies between the force and the resistance. An example is the skull pivoting on the atlas with the weight of the head held by the trapezius and sternocleidomastoid muscles.

- Second-class lever — The resistance lies between the fulcrum and the point of effort. An example is the gastrocnemius and soleus muscles lifting the body's weight by acting through the ball of the foot.
- Third-class lever — The effort lies between the resistance and the fulcrum. An example is the action of the biceps lifting a load held in the hand through bending the elbow.

Muscles and Nerves of the Pectoral Girdle

The *pectoralis major* originates in the clavicular head-medial half of the clavicle, the sternocostal head-anterior sternum, and the aponeurosis of the external oblique. It inserts on the lateral lip of the intertubercular groove of the humerus and covers the upper thorax. It is innervated by the lateral and medial pectoral nerves (C5, C6, C7, C8, and T1), and adducts and medially rotates the humerus. The *pectoralis minor* originates near the costal cartilages of ribs 3 to 5, and inserts on the coracoid process of the scapula. It is covered by the *pectoralis major* and innervated by the medial pectoral nerve (C8 and T1). The *serratus anterior* lies in the lateral thorax. It originates from the lateral parts of ribs 1 through 8, inserts on the scapula, and is innervated by the long thoracic nerves (C5, C6, and C7). It protracts the scapula and secures it to the body. Other muscles indirectly involved in minor movements of the pectoral girdle are the *subclavius*, the *levator scapulae*, the *rhomboideus*, and the *trapezius*.

Extrinsic (Superficial) Muscles of the Back

The trapezius muscle attaches the pectoral girdle to the skull and vertebral column. It also elevates, lowers, retracts, and rotates the scapula, and lowers the shoulder. The *latissimus dorsi* is a wide, fan-shaped muscle connecting the thorax and the humerus. It originates from the spinous processes of the lowermost thoracic vertebrae and ribs, inserts on the humerus, and is innervated by the thoracodorsal nerve. The *levator scapulae* lies beneath the sternocleidomastoid and trapezius muscles. It originates from the transverse processes of C1 or C4, inserts on the medial border of the scapula, and is innervated by the dorsal scapular and cervical nerves. The deltoid muscle originates from the clavicle and the acromion and spine of the scapula, inserts on the deltoid tuberosity of the humerus, and is innervated by the axillary nerve. Together with the *pectoralis major* and coracobrachialis muscles, it abducts, flexes, extends, and rotates the humerus, and also stabilizes the shoulder joint.

Rotator Cuff Muscles

The four rotator cuff muscles—the *supraspinatus*, the *infraspinatus*, the *teres minor*, and the *subscapularis*—and their tendons attach the scapula to the humerus. As a group, they keep the humeral head in the glenoid fossa of the scapula and stabilize the shoulder joint. One or more of the rotator cuff tendons are often torn during repetitive athletic activity or as a result of simple wear and tear, resulting in pain and restricted shoulder movement.

Hip Joints

The wedge-shaped sacrum consists of five fused bones. It stabilizes the pelvis and transmits the body's weight to the pelvic girdle. It is attached to each ilium by a strong, weight-bearing synovial joint (the sacroiliac joint) and the interosseus and posterior sacroiliac ligaments, which are the strongest ligaments in the body. The two pubic bones are joined anteriorly at the pubic symphysis, a non-moving, thick cartilaginous joint reinforced by the superior pubic and arcuate pubic ligaments. The head of the femur is inserted into the cup-shaped acetabulum formed by the fusion of the ilium, the ischium, and the pubis. The entire joint is stabilized by a dense fibrous capsule surrounded by powerful muscles and ligaments.

Hip and Thigh Muscles

Hip Muscles

The anterior hip muscles are the *iliopsoas* (which includes the *psoas major*, the *iliacus*, and the *psoas minor*, the latter of which is lacking in half of the population), the *tensor fasciae latae*, the *sartorius*, and the *quadriceps femoris*. The posterior dorsal hip muscles consist of the *gluteus maximus*, the *gluteus medius*, the *gluteus minimus*, and the *piriformis*. The ventral hip muscles include the *obturator internus* and *obturator externus*, the *inferior gemellus* and *superior gemellus*, and the *quadratus femoris*. The posterior thigh (hamstring) muscles are the *semitendinosus*, the *semimembranosus*, and the *biceps femoris*.

Actions

The iliopsoas muscles are the strongest thigh flexors, and also flex the trunk from supine to sitting position. The *tensor fasciae latae* tightens the deep *fascia lata* and the iliotibial tract, enabling the gluteus maximus to keep the knee extended. The sartorius muscle runs along the adductor canal and covers the femoral artery. It flexes, abducts, and rotates the thigh laterally, flexes the leg at the knee joint, and flexes and rotates the trunk. The *quadriceps femoris*, the largest muscle (actually four muscles acting together) in the body, extends the leg and forms the quadriceps tendon that surrounds and attaches to the patella and then the tibia. The hamstring muscles (the *semitendinosus*, the *semimembranosus*, and the *biceps femoris*) both extend the thigh and flex the knee, but not simultaneously.

Innervation

All of the major hip and thigh muscles are innervated via the ventral rami of spinal nerves. The *iliopsoas* is innervated by the L1, L2, and L3 nerves; the *tensor fasciae latae* is innervated by the L4 and L5 nerves; the sartorius is innervated by the L2 and L3 nerves; the *quadriceps femoris* is innervated by the femoral nerve arising from the L2, L3, and L4 nerves; the *gluteus maximus* is innervated by the inferior gluteal nerve; the *piriformis* is innervated by the S1 and S2 nerves; and the hamstrings are innervated by the L5, S1, and S2 nerves.

Appendicular Skeleton

Limbs, including their girdles, associated ligaments, and synovial membranes, are formed from myotomes in the somatic mesoderm. The long bones develop as endochondral (cartilage replacement) bone. Unlike the other bones of the appendicular skeleton, the clavicles and scapulae are derived from dermatomes. They exhibit membranous (dermal bone) ossification first, and endochondral ossification later. They are usually classified as dermal bone.

Circulation

Deoxygenated blood carries CO_2 and cellular wastes to the right atrium of the heart through the superior and inferior *venae cavae*. It enters the right ventricle, and is pumped through the pulmonary arteries to the lungs, where CO_2 is exchanged for inspired O_2. Freshly oxygenated blood passes through the pulmonary veins into the left atrium and right ventricle, and is sent out through the aorta to all parts of the body via the subclavian and carotid arteries (upper body) and the descending aorta (lower body). The oxygenated blood travels to the viscera through the mesenteric artery, to the kidneys through the renal arteries, and to the lower trunk and legs through the common iliac artery. Spent blood is brought back to the heart from the lower body by the inferior vena cava. Blood from the intestines goes through the hepatic portal vein to the liver, where the products of digestion are processed. From the liver, spent blood passes through the hepatic vein and into the inferior vena cava, and then back to the heart.

Arteries and Veins

With just two exceptions, arteries carry oxygenated blood from the heart to the rest of the body; veins carry spent, deoxygenated blood laden with the metabolic wastes from the peripheral tissues back to the heart. The sole exceptions are the umbilical vein, which carries fresh blood from the maternal placenta to the developing fetus during fetal circulation, and the pulmonary arteries and veins. The pulmonary arteries carry spent blood from the heart to the lungs, and the pulmonary veins carry freshly oxygenated blood from the lungs back to the heart. Unlike the veins, arteries contain a prominent layer of smooth muscle cells known as the *tunica media*, which assists in moving the blood through the body against the friction of the arterial walls. The thinner tunica media of the veins does not do this. Movement of blood through the veins is assisted by the contraction of skeletal muscles during normal activity, and backflow is prevented by a series of one-way valves.

Heart

The heart is composed primarily of cardiac muscle enclosed in a double-layered pericardial sac. The wall of the heart consists of three layers: (1) an outer epicardium, which is also the inner wall of the pericardium; (2) a middle myocardium, which is composed of thick muscle that contracts spontaneously; and (3) an inner endocardium that is in direct contact with the blood. The four-chambered heart has two atria, which receive blood. The atria are located above the two ventricles, which contract and discharge the blood. Deoxygenated blood enters the right atrium from the *vena cava* and passes into the right ventricle through the tricuspid valve. Deoxygenated blood is then pumped to the lungs, where it becomes oxygenated and returns to the left atrium via the pulmonary veins. It then passes into the left ventricle through the mitral (bicuspid) valve. This completes the pulmonary circuit. The systemic circuit involves pumping the newly oxygenated blood from the left ventricle out through the aorta to all parts of the body. Semilunar valves prevent backflow of the blood from the pulmonary arteries and the aorta into their respective ventricles.

Lymph Nodes

Lymph nodes act as lymph filters. It is in the lymph nodes where macrophages destroy microbes and other foreign bodies, and also help to activate the humoral and cell-mediated immune responses. Each bean-shaped node is enclosed in a fibrous capsule. Inward-projecting trabeculae divide each node into compartments. The outer cortex contains a number of lymph follicles (nodules), which often have germinal centers with actively dividing B lymphocytes. The deeper cortex contains T lymphocytes, which perform a surveillance role as they travel between the blood, lymph, and lymph nodes. Lymph enters the node through afferent vessels, and percolates through a system of subcapsular and medullary sinuses before exiting through the efferent vessels located at the hilum.

Typical lymph node:

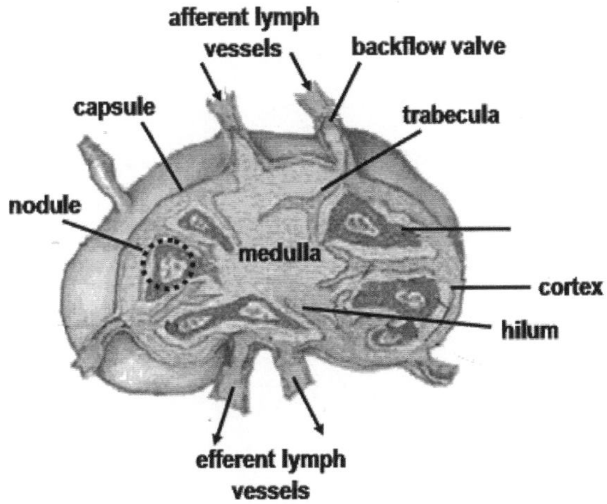

Spleen, Thymus Gland, Tonsils, and Peyer's Patches

The fist-sized spleen is located in the upper left quadrant of the abdominal cavity, below the diaphragm. It breaks down hemoglobin from senescent erythrocytes into amino acids and bilirubin, stores red blood cells and platelets, and serves as a site for lymphocyte proliferation. The thymus gland plays a role in T lymphocyte maturation, and secretes thymosin and thymopoietin that cause T cells to become immunocompetent. The paired pharyngeal tonsils (adenoids) and lingual tonsils in the pharynx gather and remove ingested and inhaled pathogens. Structurally similar to tonsils, Peyer's patches are small clusters of lymphoid follicles in the wall of the ileum which destroy bacterial pathogens in the intestine.

Lymphatic System

Lymphatic vessels develop from lymph sacs derived from vascular mesoderm. They arise first as paired sacs at the junction of the internal jugular and subclavian veins, and give rise to the lymphatic capillary plexuses throughout the thorax, the head and neck, and the arms. The retroperitoneal lymph sac forms in the intestinal mesentery of the intestine from the primitive vena cava and mesonephric veins. From here, lymphatic vessels and capillaries spread to the viscera and the diaphragm. Paired posterior lymph sacs arise from the iliac veins and produce the lymphatic capillaries and vessels of the lower abdomen, the pelvis, and the legs.

Major Visceral Organs

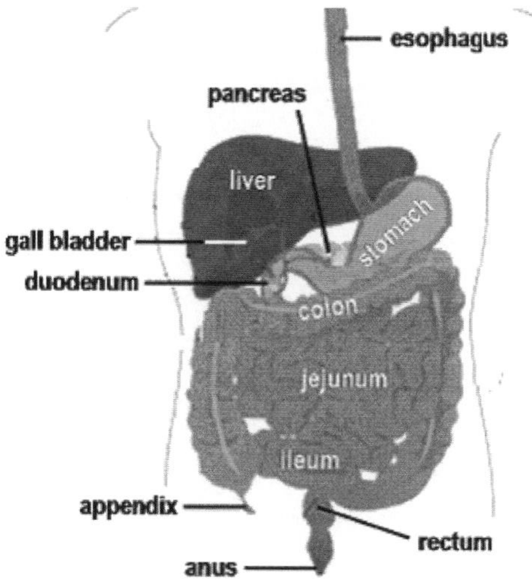

Oral Cavity and Pharynx

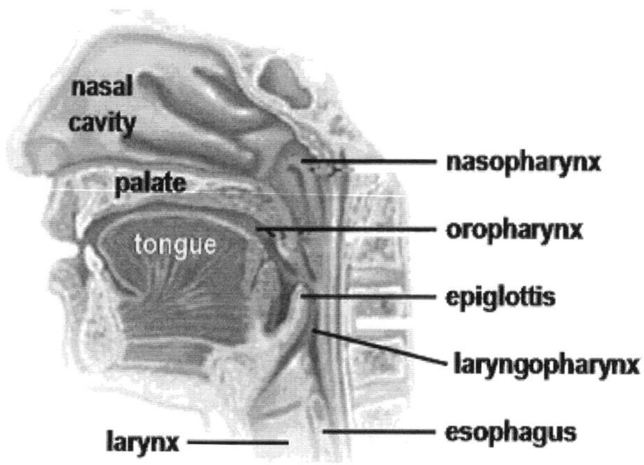

Visceral Mesenteries

The abdominal viscera include the stomach, the intestines, the liver and biliary system, the pancreas, the spleen, the kidneys, the ureters, and the suprarenal glands. The stomach and most of the intestines are fixed to the body wall by the peritoneal mesentery. The paired kidneys, the suprarenal glands, and the pancreas are retroperitoneal.

Peritoneal Suspensions of the Viscera

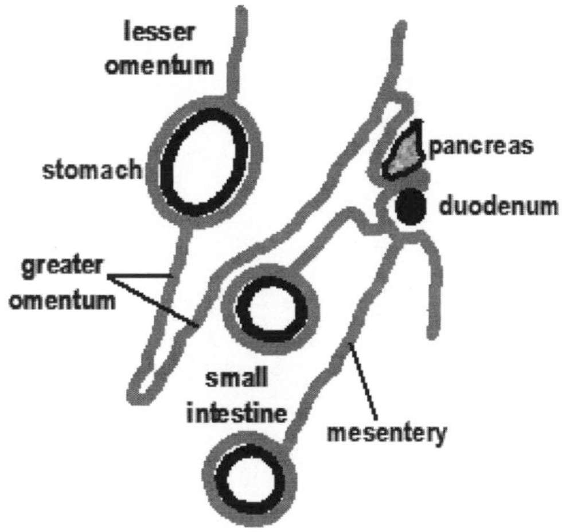

Liver

The liver is the body's largest glandular organ, and has a mass of about 1.4 kg. It is where detoxification of xenobiotics and toxic metabolites takes place. It is also the site of plasma protein, cholesterol, urea, bile, and lymph synthesis, as well as hormone production. The liver is also where aged red blood cells are destroyed and bilirubin is conjugated to glucuronic acid or sulfate and eliminated in the bile. The liver receives blood directly from the gut, which contains the products of food digestion. This blood is passed from the hepatic portal vein into an intricate system of liver sinuses, where it is in direct contact with the hepatocytes. After passage through the liver, the blood is collected in the hepatic vein and passed to the inferior vena cava for delivery to the right atrium of the heart.

Respiratory System

The human respiratory system includes the external and internal nares, the larynx, the trachea, the bronchi, the lungs and surrounding pleura, and the diaphragm and respiratory muscles. Functionally, the respiratory system consists of the respiratory zone where gas is exchanged (the respiratory bronchioles, alveolar ducts, and alveoli) and the conducting zone, which refers to all of the other passageways through which air flows to and from the respiratory zone.

Review Video: Respiratory System
Visit mometrix.com/academy and enter code: 783075

Main structures of the respiratory system:

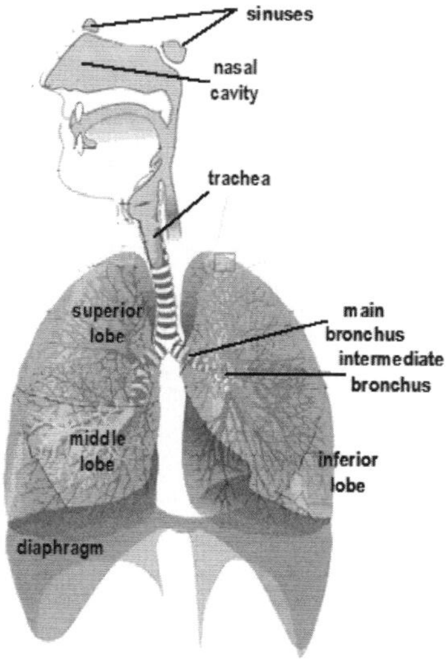

Pulmonary Alveoli

Alveoli are outcroppings of the alveolar ducts and alveolar sacs, and are the dead ends of the respiratory tree. Human lungs contain between 240 and 790 million alveoli, which provide a surface area of 70 square meters or more for gas exchange. They are grouped together in alveolar sacs that resemble clusters of interlinked grapes. They are densely surrounded by capillaries, a feature that allows for efficient gas exchange. Their thin walls secrete a surfactant to lower the surface tension of the alveolar fluid. This prevents the alveoli from collapsing due to the hydrogen bonds and other intermolecular forces binding water molecules together.

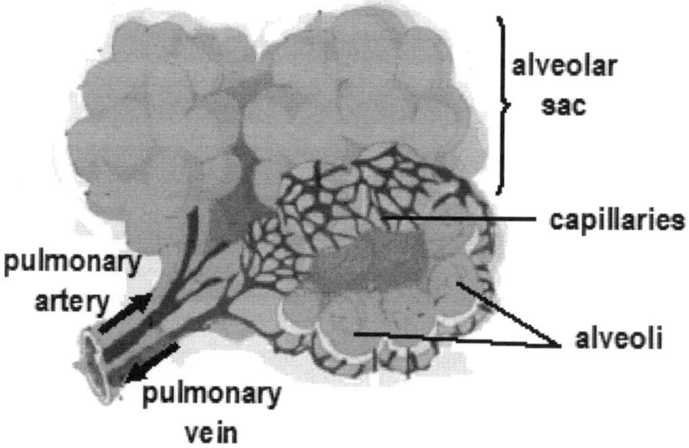

Urogenital System

The kidneys and other urinary structures and the reproductive system are derived from intermediate mesoderm. The primitive embryonic structures include the pronephros, the mesonephros and metanephros of the kidneys and ureters, and the reproductive structures. The gonads develop in place of the pronephros and mesonephros, which arise and disappear early in embryogenesis. The *vasa deferentia*, the *epididymis*, the *ducti deferentes*, the seminal vesicles, and the ejaculatory duct develop from the Wolffian ducts (pronephros) in males, while the Müllerian ducts atrophy. The oviducts and fallopian tubes arise from the Müllerian ducts (mesonephros) in females, while the Wolffian ducts disappear. The lower (caudad) portions of the Müllerian ducts fuse to form the uterus and the vagina. The kidneys develop from those portions of the metanephros that persist, while the gonads form from the peritoneum.

Reproductive Structures

Development of the reproductive structures:

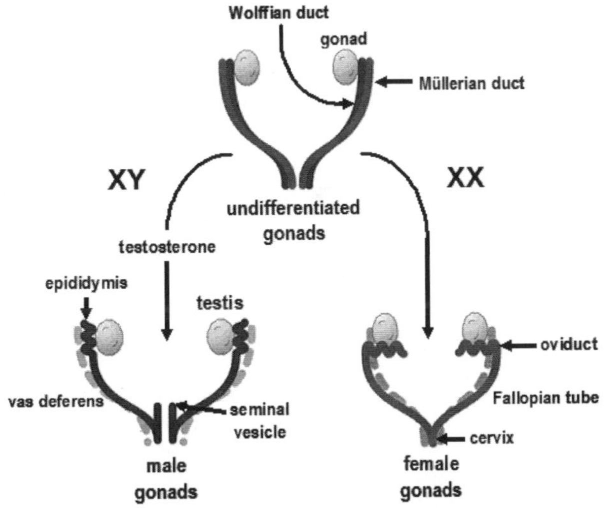

Review Video: Reproductive Systems
Visit mometrix.com/academy and enter code: 505450

Graafian Follicle

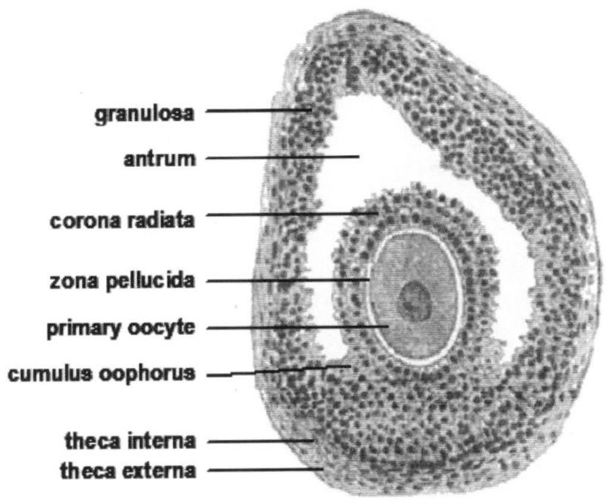

SEMINIFEROUS TUBULE

Cross section of a seminiferous tubule:

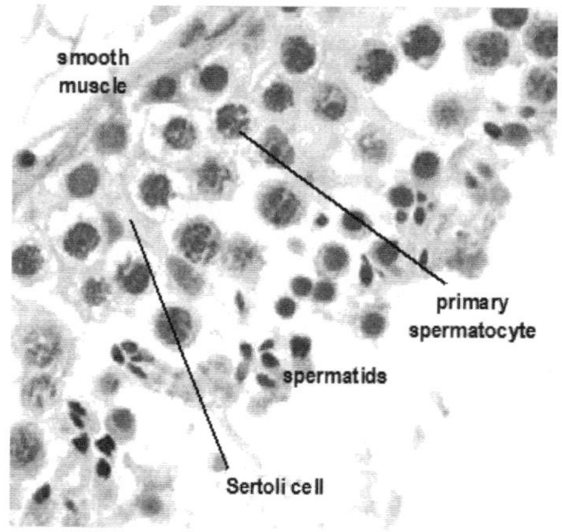

AMINE HORMONES

With the exception of thyroid hormone receptors, the receptors for amine and peptide hormones are located in the plasmalemma. All are G protein-coupled receptors that bind their ligand outside the cell and transmit a signal to a G protein complex inside the cell membrane. Epinephrine can bind to β-, α_1-, and α_2-adrenergic receptors. Norepinephrine binds mainly to α receptors. Different G proteins have distinctive α subunits that initiate separate second messenger signaling pathways: cAMP, Ca^{2+}, inositol triphosphate (IP_3), and diacylglycerol (DAG). Each type of receptor is coupled to a different G protein that activates a different signal transduction cascade. The same hormone can produce different effects when it binds to different types of receptors. When epinephrine (EPI) attaches to an α_1- or β-adrenergic receptor, it upregulates adenylyl cyclase, which in turn increases cAMP levels. Binding of EPI to an α_2-adrenergic receptor downregulates adenylyl cyclase, thereby reducing cAMP levels.

HORMONES PRODUCED BY THE STOMACH

Distension of the stomach by food stimulates G cells in the gastric pits of the antrum and adjacent duodenum to release the hormone gastrin. Gastrin release is also stimulated by gastrin-releasing peptide (GRP), which is released by the postganglionic parasympathetic fibers of the vagus nerve in response to the sight, smell, and/or thought of food. Gastrin is carried by the blood to the fundus of the stomach, where it stimulates parietal cells to secrete HCl. The increased acidity due to the release of HCl stimulates the chief cells to secrete the zymogen (prohormone) pepsinogen. HCl cleaves pepsinogen and causes it to unfold into the active protease pepsin. Increasing acidity in the stomach causes the enteric nervous system to secrete the hormone somatostatin, which inhibits further gastrin release.

ENTEROGASTRONES PRODUCED BY THE SMALL INTESTINE

The drop in pH as acidic chyme enters the small intestine causes specialized enteroendocrine S cells in the crypts of Lieberkühn in the duodenum to release secretin. Secretin is carried by the blood to the pancreas, where it causes exocrine glands to release $NaHCO_3$. The bicarbonate flows through the pancreatic duct into the duodenum, where it neutralizes the acidity of the chyme. Secretin also stimulates the bile duct cells of the gallbladder to release bile and additional bicarbonate into the small intestine. Secretin also inhibits gastrin secretion in the stomach and suppresses gastric motility. Other enterogastrones that inhibit gastric motility include somatostatin, cholecystokinin (CCK), and vasoactive intestinal peptide (VIP). Gastric inhibitory peptide (GIP) plays a minor role in this regard, but mainly directly stimulates insulin release by the pancreas through a mechanism that is not dependent on plasma glucose levels. CCK augments the effects of secretin, and causes the pancreas to release amylase, lipase, and several protease zymogens.

Melatonin

Melatonin, an indoleamine hormone derived from serotonin, is the primary hormone secreted by the pineal gland. It regulates our circadian (diurnal/nocturnal) rhythms of wakefulness and sleep. Melatonin is also involved in mediating immune and stress responses, and it plays a role in certain aspects of the aging process. Melatonin plays a major role in regulating our innate biological clock [the suprachiasmatic nucleus (SCN) in the hypothalamus], which is adjusted according to certain environmental cues, especially the intensity and duration of daylight. Bright artificial light suppresses melatonin and alters the setting of this innate clock. Under normal circumstances, melatonin levels in the blood are highest at night when we are asleep. Melatonin production ceases at dawn, and levels are at their lowest at midday.

Thymus Gland

The thymus gland produces mature T lymphocytes, which play a role in cell-mediated immunity. It secretes hormones (thymosins), which play a role in developing and maintaining normal immune responses. It is the first organ of the lymphatic system to develop in the fetus. Lymphocytes dispersed from the thymus give rise to the peripheral lymph nodes. The thymus begins to atrophy at puberty due to circulating sex hormones, and by age 75 or so is only one-sixth the size it was at puberty. Nevertheless, some level of T lymphocyte production continues throughout life. Developing hematopoietic T cells (thymocytes) undergo a complex selective process through which they develop tolerance for endogenous self-antigens and learn to recognize pathogenic foreign antigens. Only one to three percent of the thymocytes acquire the necessary immunocompetence to survive and become mature T cells. Mature T cells migrate to the spleen and peripheral lymph nodes, where they reside until they are mobilized during an immune system response.

Hormones Produced by the Heart

The heart secretes four natriuretic peptides that interact with the brain, the kidneys, and the adrenal glands to maintain Na^+, K^+, and blood volume homeostasis. The two most important of these are atrial natriuretic peptide (ANP) and brain natriuretic peptide (BNP). ANP and BNP are directly stimulated by pressure against stretch receptors in the atria of the heart. ANP is released immediately in response to increased blood volume, blood pressure, Na^+ levels, angiotensin II levels, and physical exercise, and has a circulating half-life of about one minute. BNP is typically released within an hour of cardiac overload. These hormones act on the posterior pituitary and inhibit aldosterone production. This inhibits the release of vasopressin (antidiuretic hormone) from the posterior pituitary and increases diuresis, thus lowering blood volume. Both hormones also act in the kidneys to increase the glomerular filtration rate (GFR) and inhibit the release of renin, which reduces circulating levels of angiotensin II. BNP increases vascular relaxation. All of these effects lower blood volume and pressure and increase the excretion of sodium.

Interactions Between Vitamin D and Parathyroid Hormone

Ultraviolet B radiation from sunlight converts provitamin D_3 (7-dehydrocholesterol) in the skin (*stratum basale* and *stratum spinosum*) into an inactive form of vitamin D_3, cholecalciferol. A small amount of vitamin D is also obtained from dietary sources. Cholecalciferol is carried to the liver, where it is converted into a prohormone, calcidiol (25-hydroxyvitamin D_3). Calcidiol is then carried to the kidneys, where it is converted into the active form of vitamin D_3: calcitriol. Decreased plasma levels of calcium stimulate the release of parathyroid hormone (PTH) from the parathyroid glands. PTH stimulates the conversion of calcidiol to calcitriol. Calcitriol and PTH increase calcium levels by increasing calcium resorption by the gut and kidneys and activating osteoclasts to mobilize calcium from bone and release it into the bloodstream. Calcitriol inhibits PTH release to maintain calcium levels within physiological limits.

Pituitary Hormones

The adenohypophysis (anterior pituitary) secretes six hormones. Four of these hormones are tropic hormones: somatotropic (growth) hormone (GH), thyroid-stimulating hormone (TSH), adrenocorticotropic hormone (ACTH), and the gonadotropins [follicle-stimulating hormone (FSH) and luteinizing hormone (LH)]. Gonadotropins are themselves stimulated by gonadotropin-releasing hormone secreted by the hypothalamus. The adenohypophysis also secretes β-endorphin and prolactin. Oxytocin and vasopressin are secreted by the hypothalamus and stored in the neurohypophysis (posterior pituitary). From here, they are released into the blood.

Spinal Anatomy

Superficial Muscles of the Back

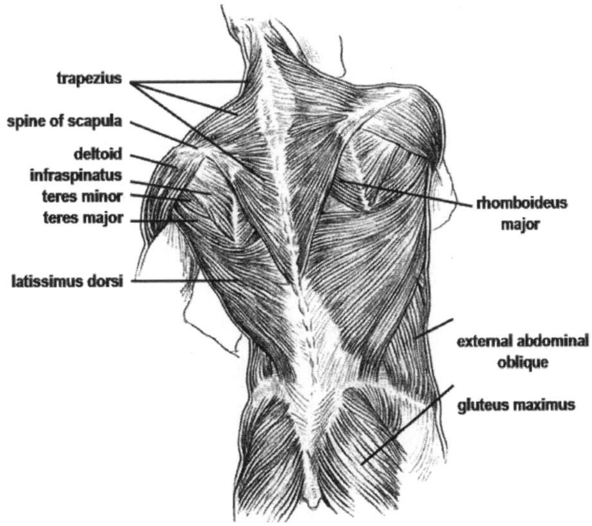

Superficial Muscles of the Anterior Thorax and Abdomen

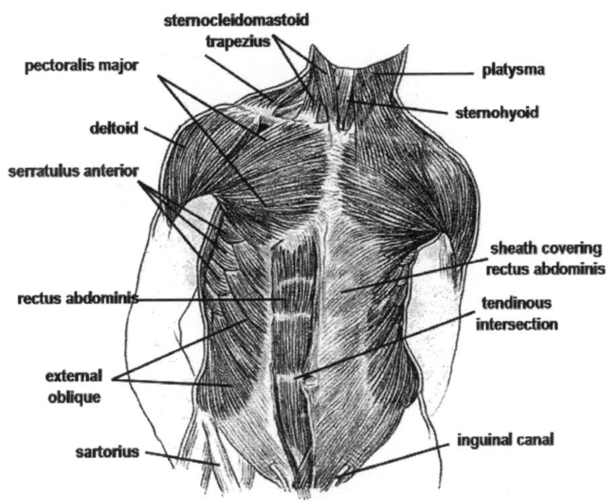

Joints

Structurally, joints are classified as fibrous, cartilaginous, and synovial. Fibrous joints are fused tightly together by dense collagenous fibers, cartilaginous joints are loosely connected by cartilage, and synovial joints (diarthroses) are highly moveable joints. The latter type is found where the cartilage-padded ends of two long bones make contact, and are secured by accessory ligaments. Functionally, joints are categorized as rigid synarthroses, such as those fusing the skull bones together; slightly moveable amphiarthroses, such as the joints between adjacent vertebrae; and highly moveable diarthroses (synovial joints). Joints may also be classified as simple (two articular surfaces), compound (three or more joining surfaces), or complex (two or more joining surfaces plus their intervening cartilage pads).

HUMAN SKULL

The skull consists of the neurocranium enclosing the brain and brainstem, and the viscerocranium comprising the face. The neurocranium usually has 8 bones (not counting the ear ossicles) and the face usually has 14, although individual variations are fairly common. Different sources give different numbers, depending on whether paired bones are counted once or twice, and on which bones are actually included. With the exception of the mandible, the bones of the skull are joined by ossified and immovable synarthrodial joints. The left and right sides of the mandible are joined by a fibrous symphysis at birth, which completely ossifies into a single bone after the first year of life. The bones of the skull are formed by a combination of both dermal and endochondral bone.

FRONTAL VIEW OF THE SKULL

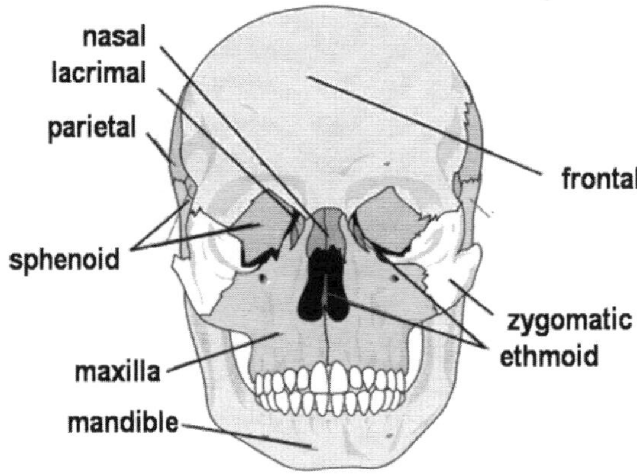

LEFT LATERAL VIEW OF THE SKULL

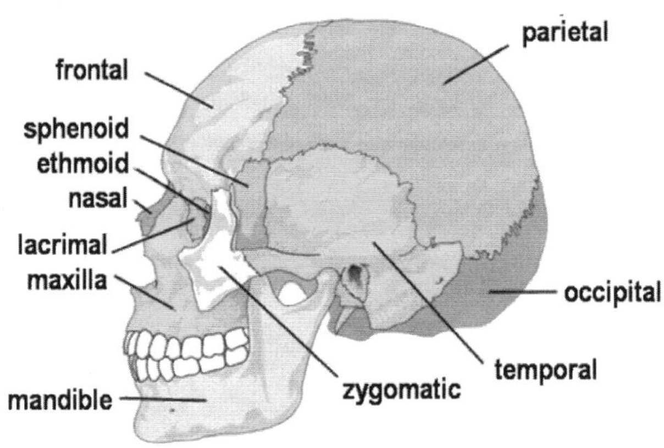

Sagittal Section of the Skull

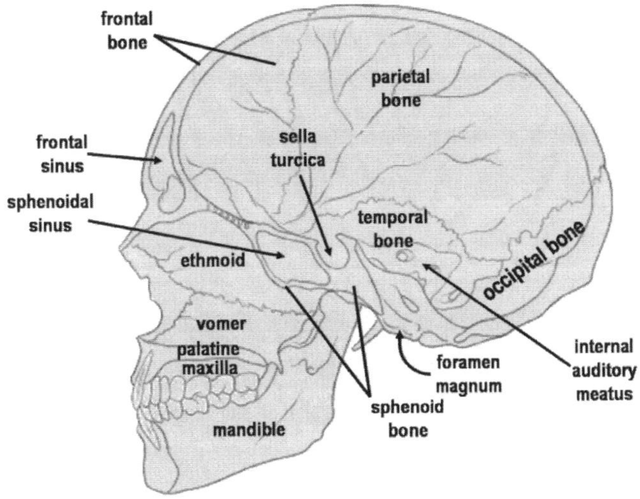

Interior Portion of the Lower Neurocranium

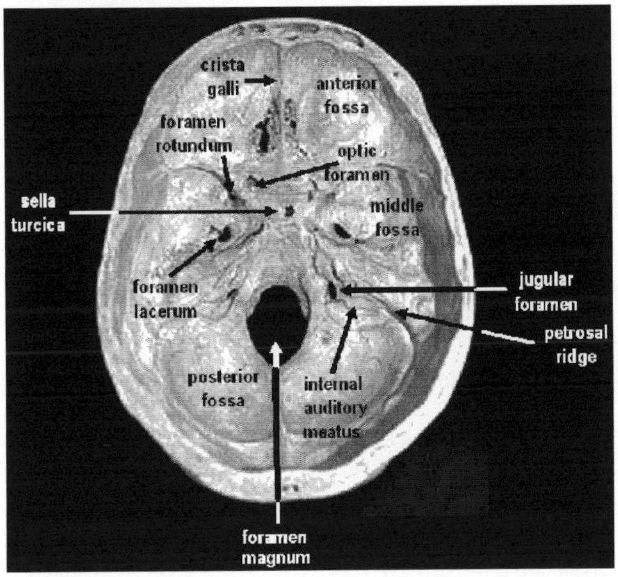

Vertebral Column

The human vertebral column typically contains 24 articulating vertebrate: 7 cervical, 12 thoracic, and 5 lumbar vertebrae (occasionally 4 or 6). The triangular, platelike sacrum usually consists of five (occasionally four or six) fused vertebrae, and the coccyx (tailbone) consists of between three and five (usually four) fused vertebrae. The upper portion of the thoracic spine is curved outward, a condition known as kyphosis, while the lumbar spine is curved inward (lordosis). The cervical vertebrae differ from all the others because they have an opening in each transverse process (the foramen transversarium) to accommodate the vertebral arteries. The skull rests and rocks forwards and backwards upon the first cervical vertebra (C1), the atlas, which lacks a body or centrum. The atlas rotates around the axis (C2). The thoracic vertebrae have facets for articulating with the heads and tubercles of the ribs. The lumbar vertebrae lack facets, and are the largest of the vertebrae. L5 connects with the underlying sacrum, which in turn is attached to the ilium on either side and to the coccyx below.

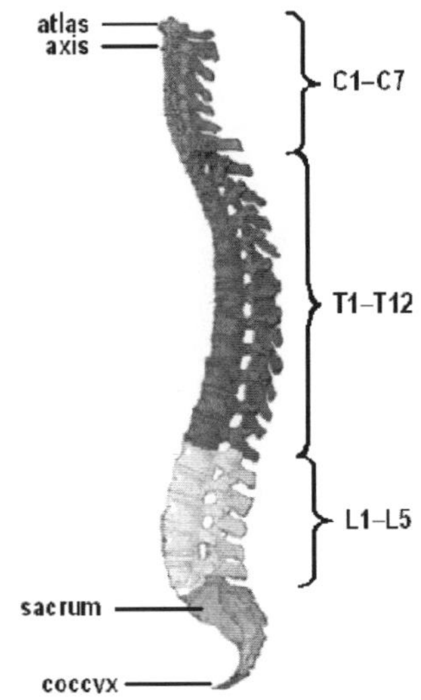

Lateral and Superior View of Thoracic Vertebra

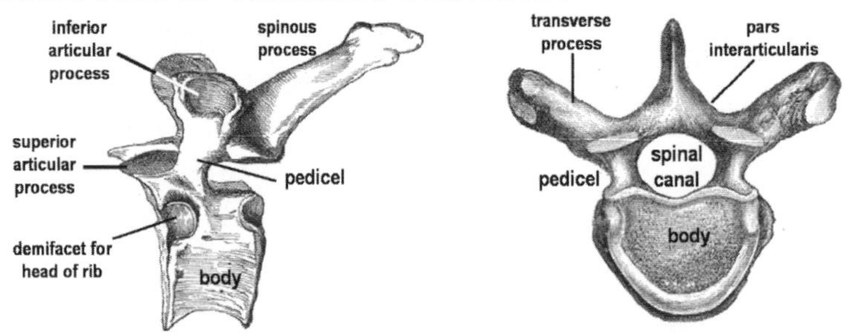

Atlas and Axis

The occipital condyles of the skull sit upon the superior articular surfaces of the uppermost cervical vertebra (C1), known as the atlas. The ring-shaped atlas is the only vertebra which lacks a vertebral body (centrum). The head can tilt up and down on the atlas. The axis, in turn, rests upon the second cervical vertebra (C2), known as the axis. The body of the axis bears a stout, upwardly direct spine called the dens (odontoid process), around which the atlas can rotate the head from side to side.

Relationship between the atlas and the axis:

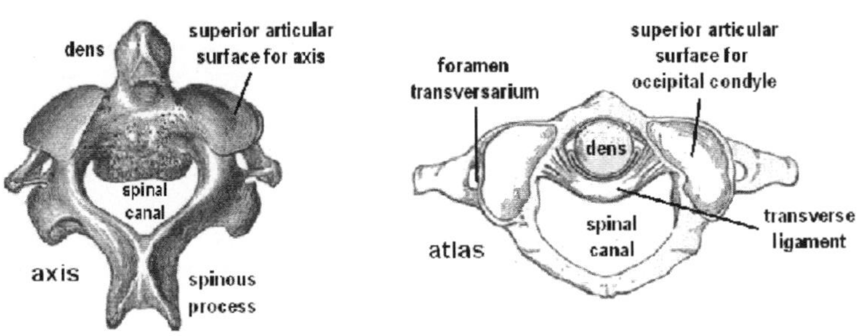

A, laterofrontal view of the atlas sitting atop the axis; B, laterofrontal aspect of the axis; C, superior aspect of the atlas and the axis:

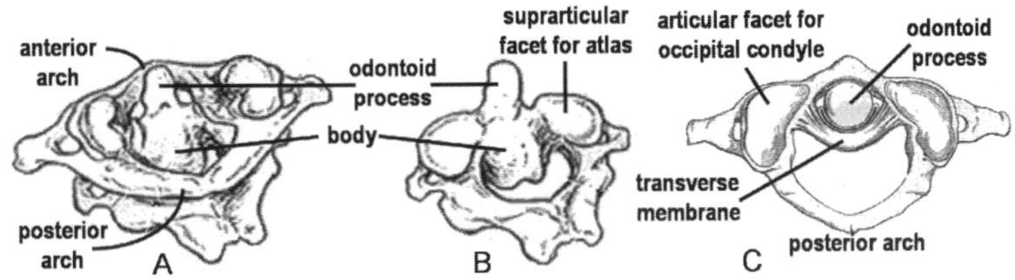

Spondylolysis and Spondylolisthesis

Spondylolysis is a congenital defect of or traumatic injury to the pars interarticularis of the vertebral arch that is found in four to six percent of the population. It is more frequently seen in young, competitive athletes because of stresses placed on the spine during sports. Obesity and lumbar lordosis are also predisposing conditions. Spondylolisthesis is a forward (anterolisthesis) or backward (retrolisthesis) displacement of a vertebra relative to the one below it. This most commonly occurs at the fourth or fifth lumbar vertebra. In children, this condition is usually the result of a congenital defect or acute trauma. In adults under age 50, it usually results from a spondylolysis. In older adults, it commonly results from degenerative disease. The X-ray image shows an anterior spondylolisthesis between L5 and S1, which is indicated by the arrow.

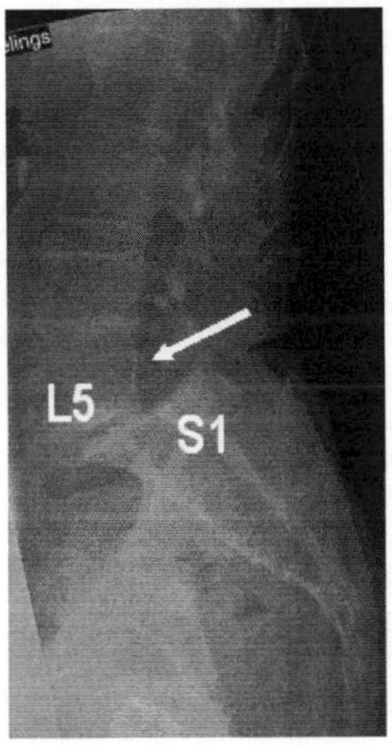

Human Ribcage and Ribs

Structure and relationship of the human ribcage and ribs:

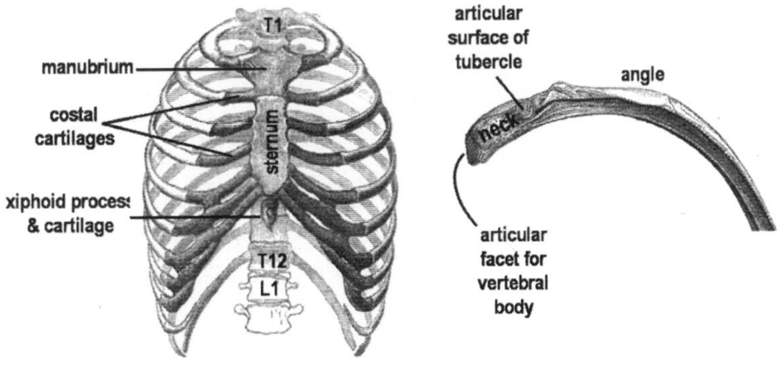

Human Pelvis

The pelvis is a basin-shaped structure formed by the two innominate (hip) bones (part of the appendicular skeleton), as well as the sacrum and the coccyx (components of the axial skeleton). Each hip bone consists of an anterior pubis and an ilium, as well as a lateroventral ischium. These bones are fused posteriorly with the sacrum and the coccyx. The articular spine sits upon S1 of the sacrum, and the head of each femur inserts into the acetabulum. In males, the pelvis is heart-shaped, and is larger and heavier than the female pelvis. The female pelvis is relatively smaller, but is wider and rounder to facilitate childbirth. There is a great deal of variation among individuals, however.

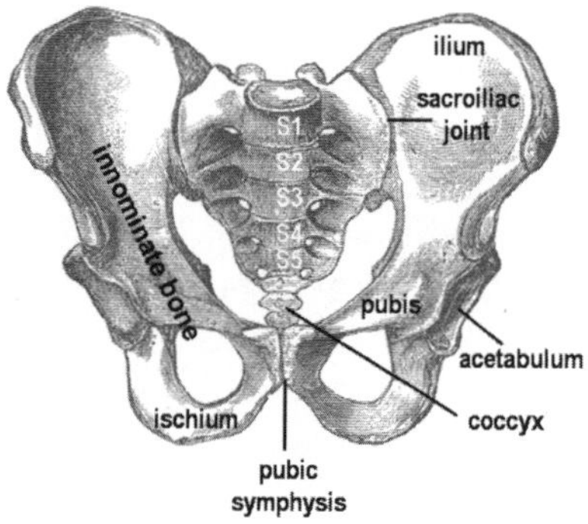

Embryonic Development of the Vertebrae

Mesodermal somites form on either side of the neural groove by week three of gestation, and differentiate into dermatomes and sclerotomes. The vertebrae develop as endochondral bone from the sclerotomes, while the vertebral body forms from the notochord. The notochord forms during gastrulation, and is the organizing center that induces formation of the neural plate and subsequent embryonic structures. The ventromedial region of each somite grows inward to surround the notochord, which differentiates into the vertebral bodies and discs. Ossification continues after birth, and is not complete until the mid-twenties.

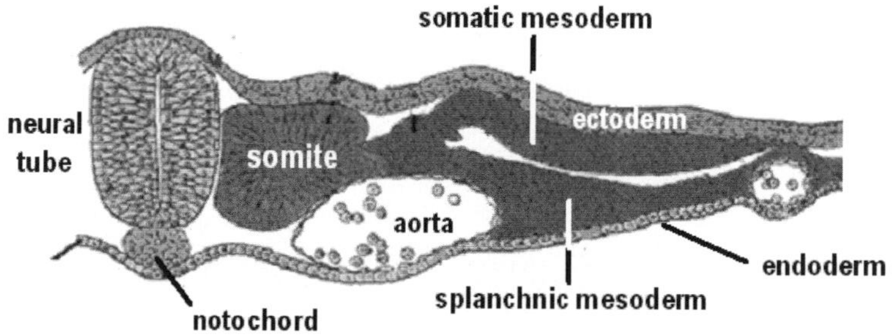

Development of the Innominate (Coxal) Bone

Each innominate bone (*os coxae*) ossifies from three primary centers for the ilium, the ischium, and the pubis. In addition, secondary centers form for the iliac crest, the anterior inferior spine, the ischial tuberosity, and a Y-shaped cartilage at the base of the acetabulum where the ilium, the ischium and the pubis merge. Ossification is not complete until about age 25.

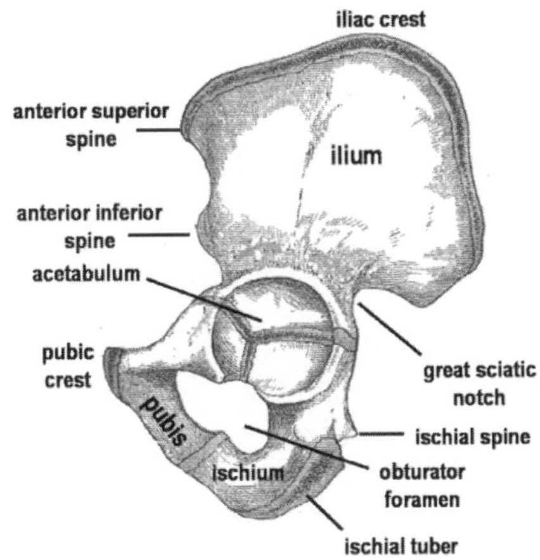

Facial Muscles

The facial muscles are superficial muscles originating on the cranial bones and inserting on the skin. They are innervated by the facial nerve (cranial nerve 7). The associated masseter and other muscles of mastication insert on the mandible, and are innervated by the trigeminal nerve (cranial nerve 5)

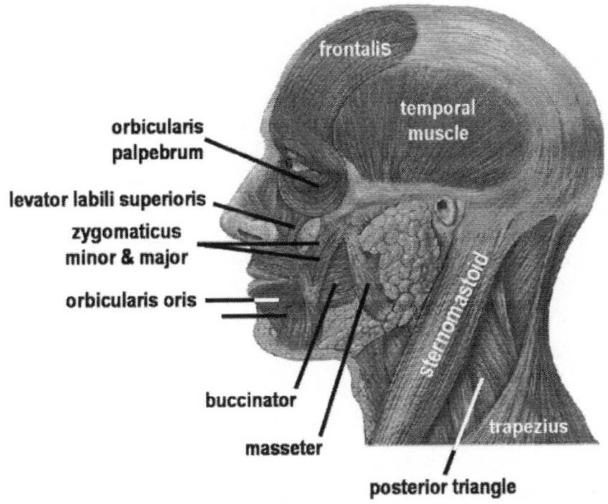

Erector Spinae and Associated Deep Muscles of the Back

The erector spinae is a bundle of three muscles—the iliocostalis, the longissimus, and the spinalis—and associated tendons lying in a groove on either side of the spine. Each of these muscles is further subdivided into three smaller muscles that vary widely in terms of size and structure depending on their position along the spinal column. The erector spinae originates from a broad aponeurosis on the sacrum, and inserts onto various thoracic and cervical vertebrae, as well as the skull. Associated muscles include the semispinalis dorsi and the multifidus, among others. Some of these are labeled in the figure on the right. Modern usage often substitutes the descriptor *thoracis* in place of *dorsi*.

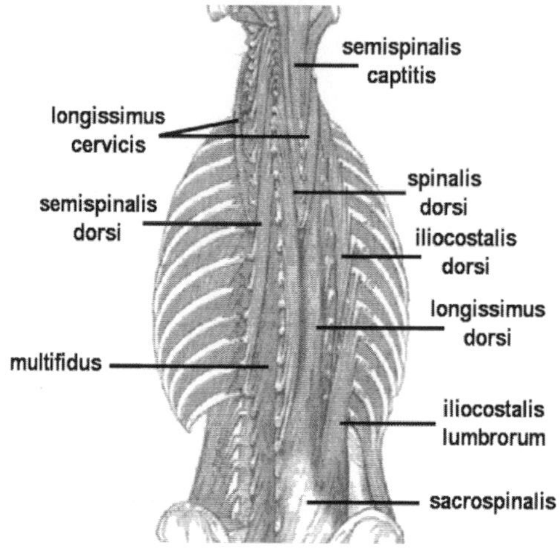

Muscles of the Neck

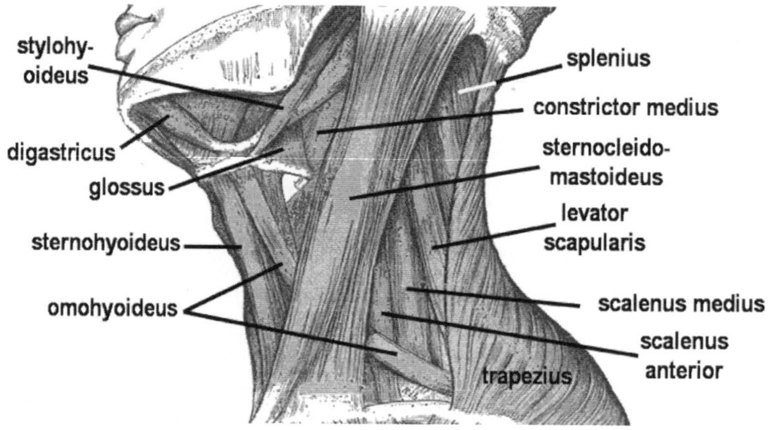

Muscles of the Perineal Region

Figure shows coronal section of male (left) and female (right) perineum:

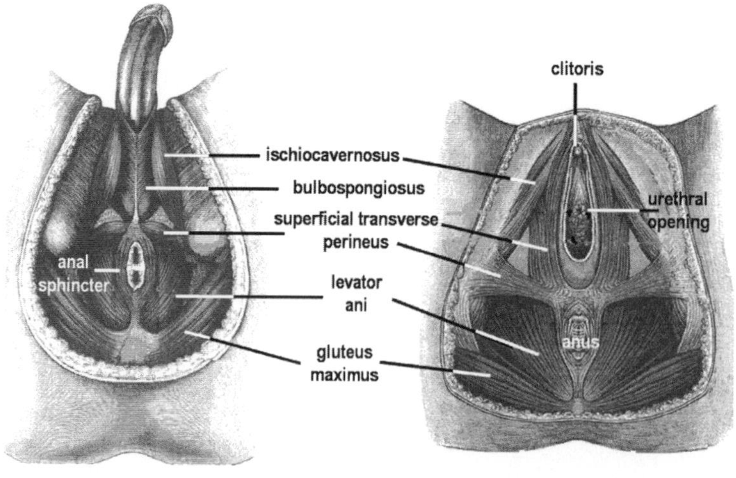

Muscles of the Pelvis

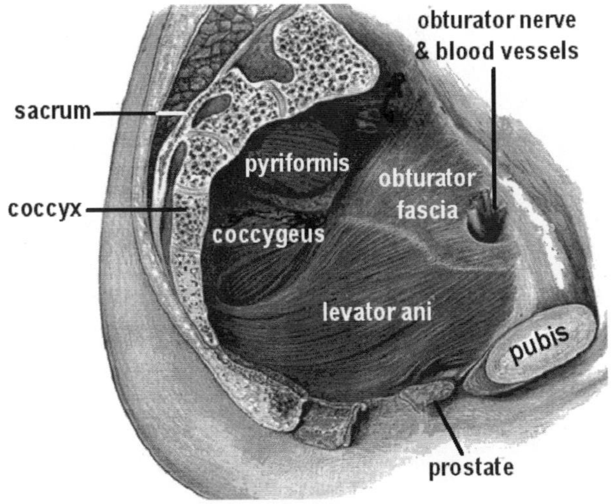

Embryonic Origin of the Axial Musculature

The axial mesoderm on either side of the notochord thickens and forms the paraxial mesoderm, which then begins to sequentially and posteriorly form segments from the anterior region. The large medial portion of each somite differentiates into the sclerotome, which will develop into the vertebrae of the spine. The dorsolateral crescent will develop into the dermomyotome, which then differentiates into the dermatome and the myotome. The dermatome will give rise to the dermis and associated structures. The myotome will give rise to the axial musculature. The myotome subsequently differentiates dorsally into the epimere (which will produce the epiaxial muscles) and ventrally into the hypomere (which will give rise to most of the muscles of the trunk and limbs).

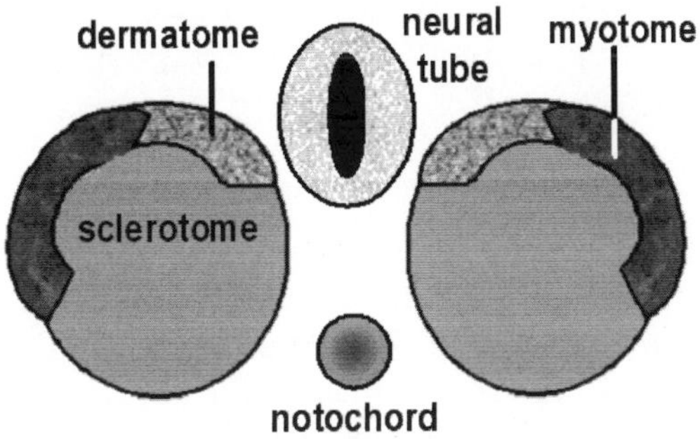

Sacroiliac Joint

The two sacroiliac (SI) joints connect the sacrum with the ilium on each side. The two irregular interlocking articular surfaces of each joint are held together by the anterior, posterior, and interosseus sacroiliac ligaments. The anterior ligament is thin and not very strong, and is sometimes described as a "slight swelling." The major support for the SI joint comes from the dorsal portion of the posterior and interosseus ligaments; the latter is stronger than the bone itself, and will not tear even if the pelvis is broken. The posterior SI ligaments consist of the short and long ligaments, which maintain the necessary balance between joint stability and flexibility.

Sacroiliac Ligaments

A, right SI ligaments, anterior view; B, right SI ligaments, posterior view:

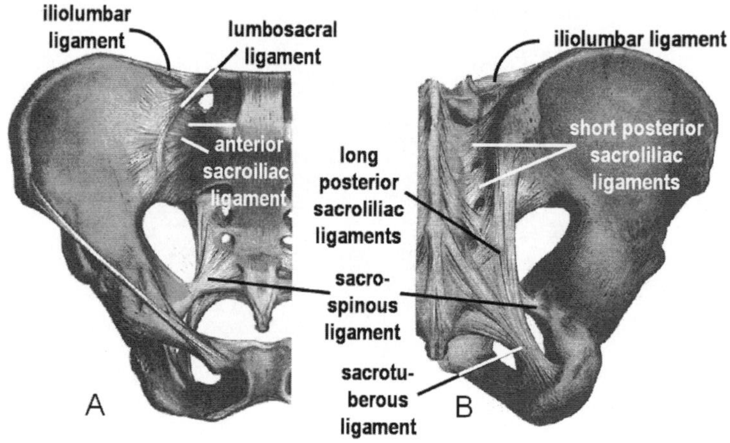

Atlantoaxis Joint

The atlantoaxial joint consists of four separate joints and their ligaments. The atlas pivots around the fingerlike odontoid process (dens) of the axis, where it is secured by the transverse membrane. This median joint consists of (a) an articulation between the posterior surface of the anterior arch and the front of the odontoid process and (b) the anterior surface of the transverse ligament and the rear of the odontoid process. Two lateral arthrodial (gliding) articulations support the lateral masses of the atlas. The apical odontoid ligament and an alar ligament on each side connect the odontoid process with the occipital bone of the skull. Loose atlantoaxial articular capsules on either side connect the margins of the atlas with the posterior articular surfaces of the axis. The strong anterior atlantoaxial ligament attaches the anterior arch of the atlas to the anterior part of the body of the axis. The posterior atlantoaxial ligament connects the posterior arch of the atlas to the laminae of the neural spine of the axis.

Injuries

The atlas is the most fragile vertebra in the spinal column. It will fracture with any displacement of the C0–C1 alignment that exceeds one millimeter. Similarly, any C1–C2 anteroposterior translation exceeding 4 millimeters, any total right and left overhang exceeding 7 millimeters, or any unilateral traumatic axial rotation exceeding 45 degrees will result in injury. The pars interarticularis and the odontoid process are the structures of the axis most likely to fail under hyperextension, but the transverse ligament is also subject to failure. The vertebral artery penetrates the posterior atlantoaxial ligament and enters the foramen magnum. This artery can be irritated or occluded by shifts in the relationships between the occiput, the atlas, and the axis. A shift of the occiput on the atlas can also produce a shift in the center of gravity that can lead to spinal scoliosis.

Biomechanics of the Vertebrae and the Intervertebral Joints

All vertebrae below C2 are functionally triaxial. The vertical axis of the posterior portion of the annulus fibrosis permits rotational motion. The anteroposterior axis running through the center of the vertebral disc allows for lateral flexion. The lateral axis in the posterior portion of the annulus fibrosis enables flexion and extension. The anterior spinal ligaments limit extension, the posterior spinal ligaments limit flexion, and the intertransverse ligaments limit bending to the opposite side around the joint's anteroposterior axis through this disc. The figure shows the ligaments of the vertebrae: 1, supraspinous ligament; 2, interspinous ligament; 3, ligamentum flavum; 4, posterior longitudinal ligament; 5, facet joint capsules; 6, intertransverse ligaments; and 7, anterior longitudinal ligament.

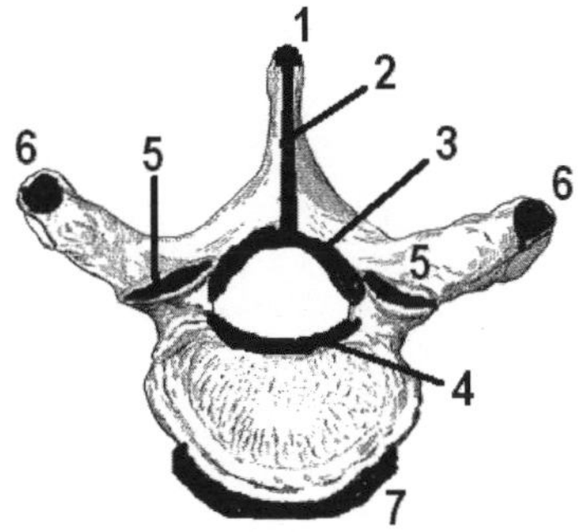

HUMAN BRAIN

The human cerebral cortex sits like a great mushroom atop the diencephalon (3rd ventricle), and the midbrain and the brainstem are beneath it. The cerebellum is located below the cerebrum on the dorsal (rear) surface of the brainstem at the level of the pons. The adult brain in males is generally larger than that of females, but this does not correlate with any differences in cognitive ability. The cerebral cortex is a thin, sheetlike layer that is two to four millimeters thick. It covers a series of deep fissures (sulci) and ridges (gyri) that produce a total surface area of 0.121 square meters, and contain some 80–120 billion neurons. Underlying the cortex is a series of myelinated tracts and neuron centers called nuclei. Each of the two cerebral hemispheres is divided into four major sections: the frontal, parietal, temporal, and occipital lobes.

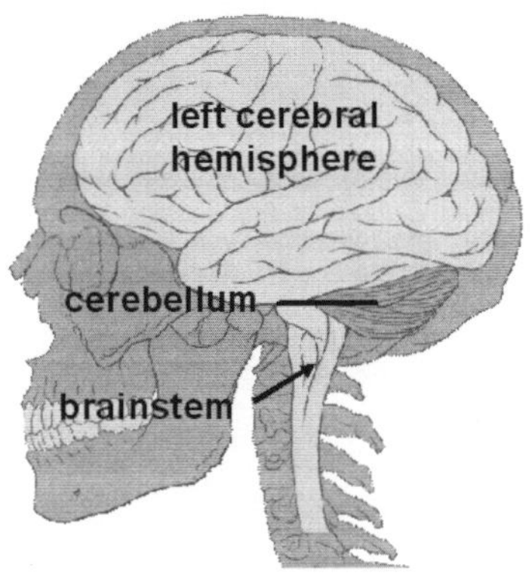

MAJOR REGIONS

Each cerebral hemisphere is divided into a frontal lobe, a parietal lobe, a temporal lobe, and an occipital lobe. The frontal lobe is involved with reasoning, movement, logic, problem solving, and abstract thinking. It is separated from the parietal lobe by the fissure of Rolando (central sulcus). The parietal lobe integrates sensory input, and is involved in spatial orientation and navigation. It is separated from the temporal lobe by the fissure of Sylvius (lateral fissure). The temporal lobe receives auditory input and functions in semantics; it includes the hippocampus, and is also involved in memory. The occipital lobe is associated with vision. The cerebellum is involved in the coordination, precision, and fine tuning of movements initiated from the higher cortical centers of the brain.

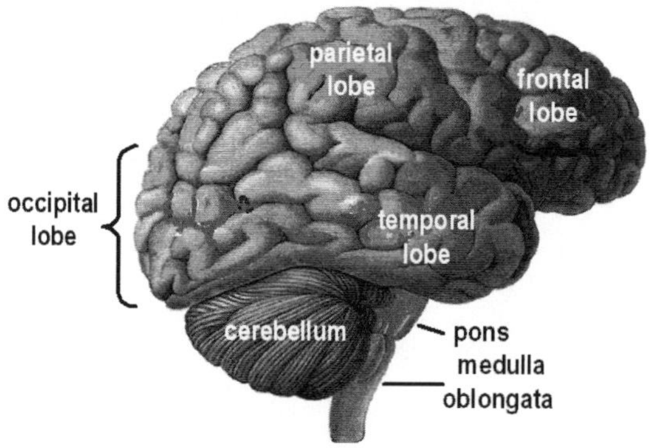

Cranial Nerves

The 12 cranial nerves emerge directly from the brain. The first two derive from the cerebrum, while the rest come out of the brainstem. In order, they are I, olfactory; II, optic; III, oculomotor; IV, trochlear; V, trigeminal; VI, abducens; VII, facial; VIII, auditory (vestibulocochlear); IX, glossopharyngeal; X, vagus; XI, spinal accessory; and XII, hypoglossal. They are named according to their function. A classical mnemonic device for remembering the sequence is based on the first letter of each nerve: "On old Olympus' towering tops, a Finn and German viewed some hops."

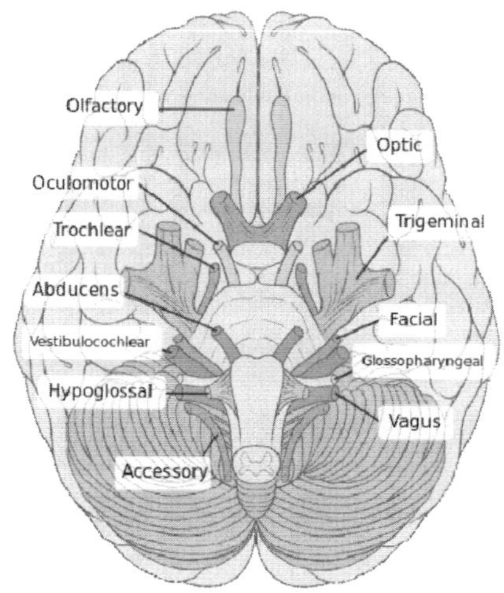

Meninges

The meninges are a series of three membranes that enclose the central nervous system (i.e. both the brain and the spinal cord). Arranged from the outermost position to the innermost, they are the dura mater, the arachnoid, and the pia mater. The dura mater is the thickest, toughest, and most fibrous of the three layers. The falx cerebri, a prominent infolding, separates the cerebral hemispheres. The arachnoid mater is the thin, delicate middle layer. Except for the longitudinal fissure between the two hemispheres, it does not follow the brain's contours, and encloses it like a loose sack. It is separated from the pia mater by the cerebrospinal fluid (CSF)-filled subarachnoid space. The CSF is produced by the choroid plexus. The innermost pia mater is a very thin and delicate membrane that closely follows the brain's gyri and sulci. The arachnoid and pia mater are collectively called the leptomeninges, and form the blood-brain barrier. These same three layers also enclose the spinal cord.

Cranial meninges and their associated structures:

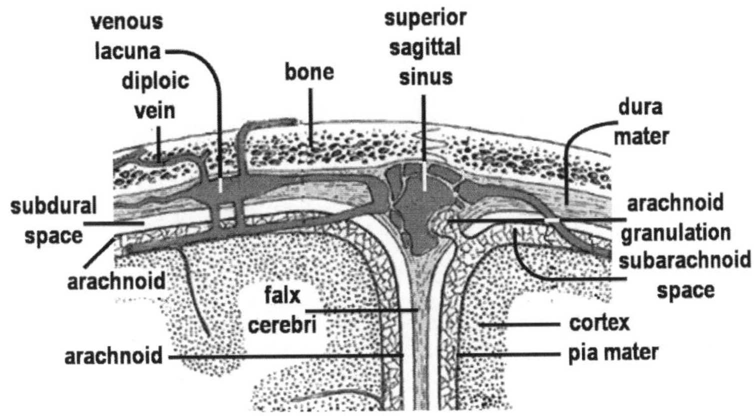

Meninges:

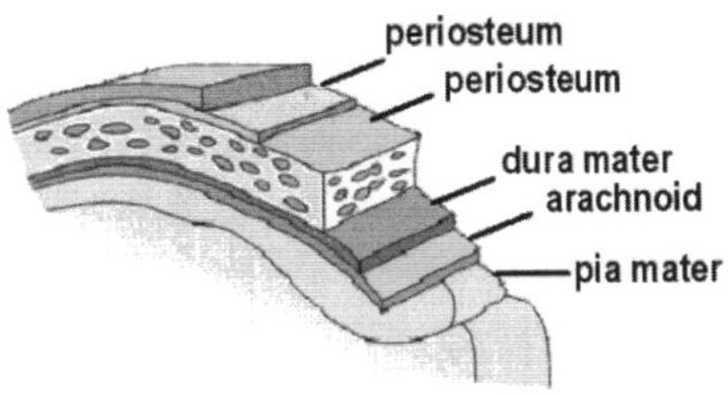

Circulation to the Brain

The brain is supplied by the paired carotid and vertebral arteries. The external carotid arteries supply the face and superficial regions of the brain, while the internal branches and the vertebral arteries feed into the circle of Willis, which connects them with their counterparts in the opposite hemisphere. These arteries provide blood to the anterior portions of the cerebral hemispheres, along with their white matter and basal ganglia. The posterior and medial portions of the hemispheres, the diencephalon, the cerebellum, and the brainstem are supplied by the paired vertebral arteries, which fuse into the basilar artery before joining the circle of Willis. The brain is drained through a series of superficial dural venous sinuses in the dura mater, which eventually empty into the two jugular veins.

Major Arteries to the Brain

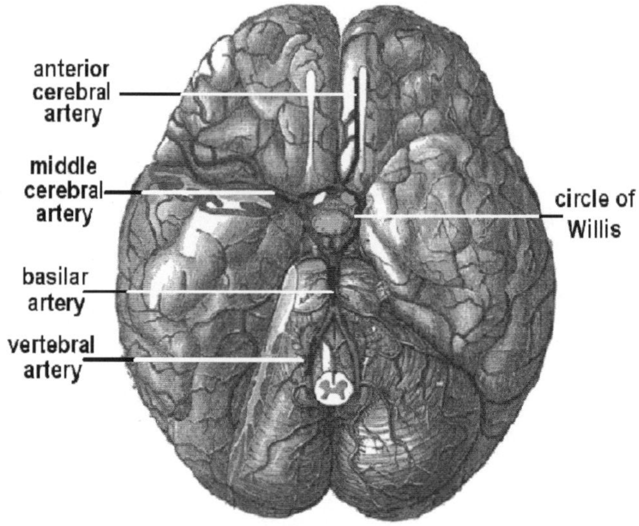

Ventricles of the Brain

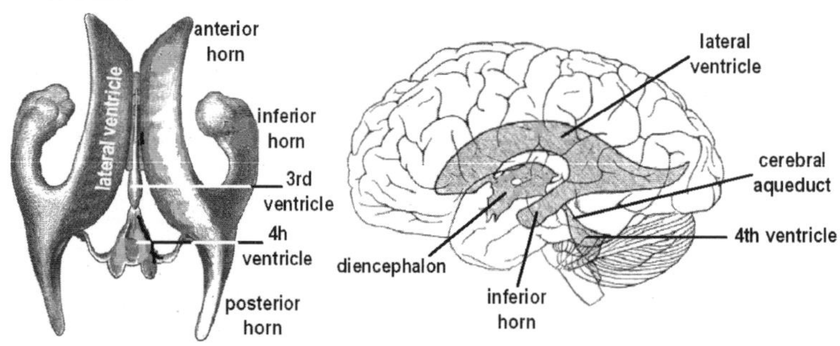

The brain has four ventricles, which are continuous with the spinal canal. The first two ventricles are the left and right lateral ventricles, respectively. Together, they form the telencephalon and develop into the two cerebral hemispheres. The first two ventricles along with the third ventricle, or diencephalon, constitute the forebrain (prosencephalon). The diencephalon gives rise to the thalamus, the epithalamus, the hypothalamus, the pineal gland, and associated structures. The third ventricle is connected to the fourth ventricle lying within the pons by the cerebral aqueduct (aqueduct of Sylvius). The roof of the fourth ventricle consists of the cerebellum, and the walls are formed by the cerebellar peduncles.

Formation of the Neural Tube

The notochord, which forms during gastrulation, induces the differentiation of the neural plate from the overlying ectoderm. This neural plate then thickens and develops neural folds down its length on either side. These neural folds subsequently converge and fuse to form a hollow neural tube that runs most of the length of the developing embryo. This will become the central nervous system. The neural tube soon develops four major regions. From front to rear, these are the prosencephalon, the mesencephalon, the rhombencephalon, and the spinal cord. Multipotent neural crest cells pinch off from the neural crests and migrate to various parts of the embryo, where they give rise to melanocytes; some cartilage and bones of the face and head; smooth muscle; glial cells;

neurons of the peripheral, autonomic, and enteric nervous systems; adrenal medullae; and other tissues.

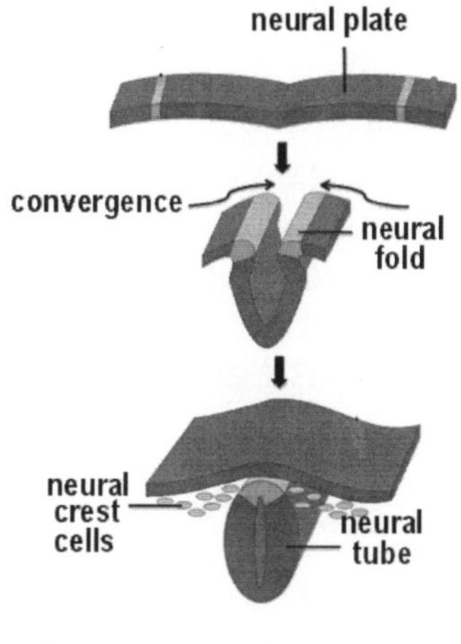

Further Differentiation of the Brain

As development proceeds, the prosencephalon forms two lateral ventricles, the telencephalon, and an undivided chamber just behind the telencephalon called the diencephalon. The two lateral ventricles of the telencephalon will become the cerebral hemispheres, while the diencephalon will give rise to the paired thalami, the epithalamus, the pineal body, the hypothalamus, and associated structures. The dorsal telencephalon (pallium) becomes the cerebral cortex, while the ventral telencephalon (subpallium) develops into the basal ganglia. The mesencephalon will develop into the midbrain, while the rhombencephalon forms the metencephalon and the myelencephalon. These develop into the pons and the cerebellum, and the medulla oblongata, respectively.

Differentiation of the brain:

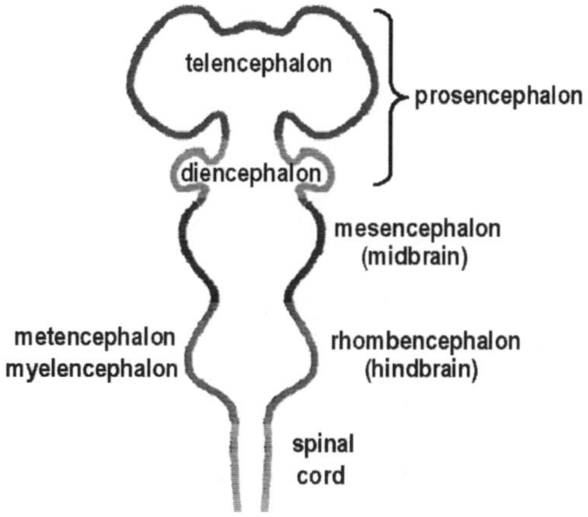

Brain Cells

The 50 to 100 or so billion neurons in the brain comprise less than 10 percent of the total number of brain cells. The rest are supporting glial cells. Unlike most neurons, glial cells are capable of mitosis. Astrocytes are important in clearing neurotransmitters from the synapse following an action potential. Oligodendrocytes are the CNS counterparts of the Schwann cells in the peripheral nervous system. Each oligodendrocyte can enclose sections of up to 50 different axons in a 1 μm-thick layer of myelin. Each Schwann cell can wrap around only a single axon segment. Microglial cells are the macrophages of the CNS, and comprise a fifth of the total glial cell population. They are the first line of defense in the immune response of the CNS, and are derived from hematopoietic stem cells from the bone marrow. Ependymal cells are ciliated, simple cuboidal epithelial cells that line the ventricles of the brain and the spinal canal. Certain ependymal cells complexed with capillaries form the choroid plexus of the brain's ventricles, which secrete the cerebrospinal fluid.

Multipolar, Bipolar, and Unipolar Neurons

Neurons fall into three major classes. Multipolar neurons have three or more dendrites that transport afferent stimuli to the cell body (soma) and a single axon. Efferent (motor) neurons are multipolar neurons. Bipolar neurons have one dendrite and one axon attached to opposite ends of the soma. They function primarily as interneurons. In unipolar or pseudounipolar neurons, which serve as afferent (sensory) neurons, the dendrite and axon emerge from a single process on the soma.

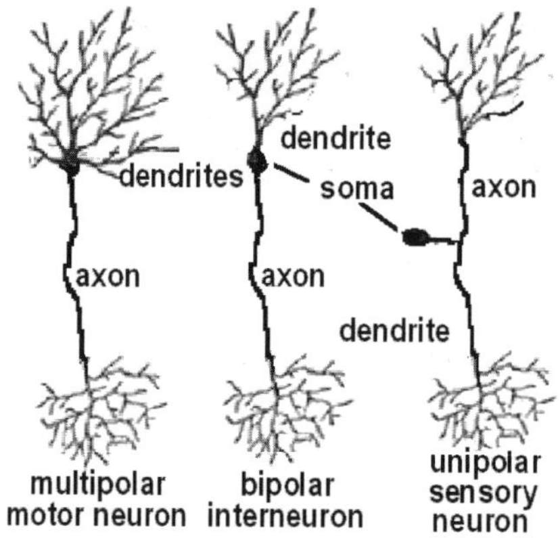

Glial Cells

Types of glial cells:

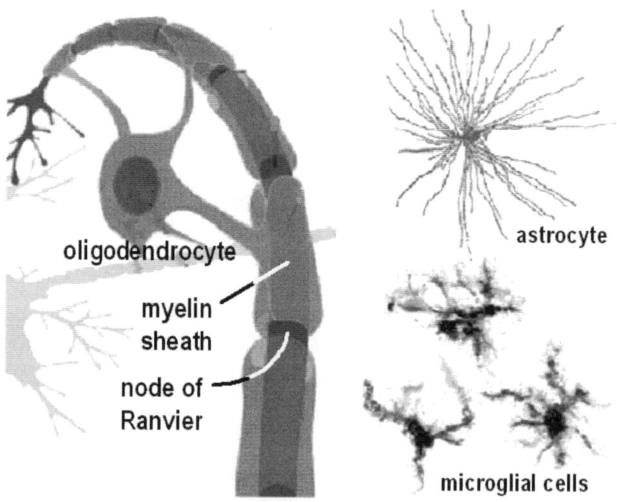

Basket, Purkinje, Granular, and Pyramidal Cells

Other specialized neurons in the brain include basket cells, Purkinje cells, granular cells, and pyramidal cells. Basket cells in the cerebral cortex and the cerebellum are interneurons that form dense networks of terminals around the somae of target cells. These inhibitory neurons release the neurotransmitter γ-aminobutyric acid (GABA). Purkinje cells are among the largest neurons in the human brain. Located in the cerebellar cortex, their dendritic trees form a dense, almost two-dimensional layer. Parallel fibers from the deeper layers pass through the dense layer comprised of the dendritic trees of Purkinje cells. Granular cells are the smallest cells in the brain. They are found in the cerebellum, the dentate gyrus of the hippocampus, and the dorsal cochlear nucleus of the olfactory bulb (cranial nerve I). They release the excitatory neurotransmitter glutamate. Pyramidal cells derive their name from their pyramid-shaped soma. They are the main excitatory neurons of the prefrontal cortex and the tracts leading from the cortex to the spinal cord.

Pyramidal, Purkinje, granular, and basket cells found in the cerebellum:

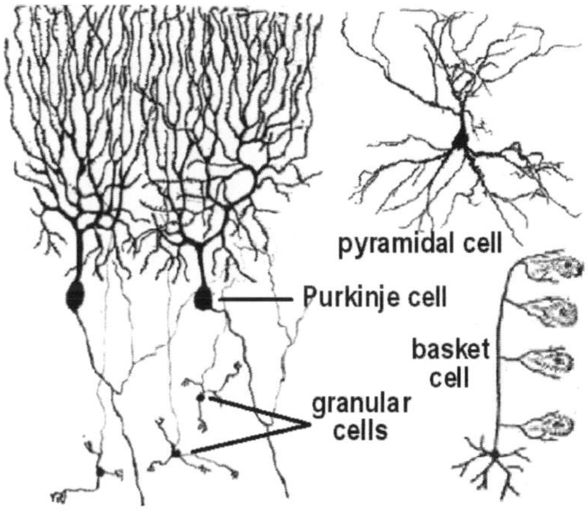

SOMATIC AND SYMPATHETIC SPINAL NEURAL CONNECTIONS

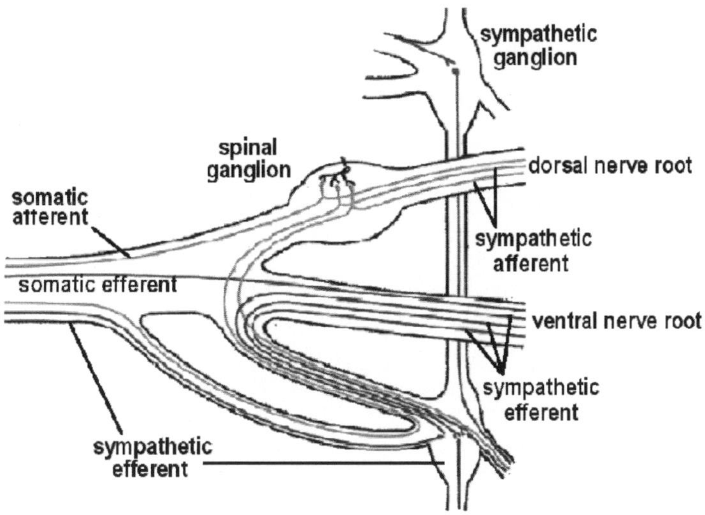

Nerves of the Brachial Plexus

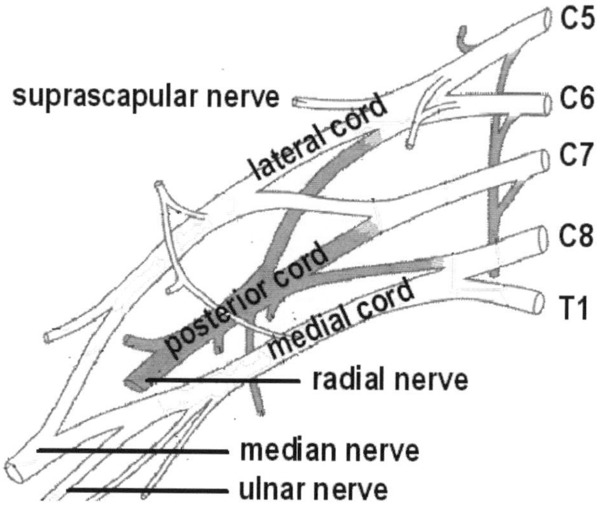

Sacral Plexus

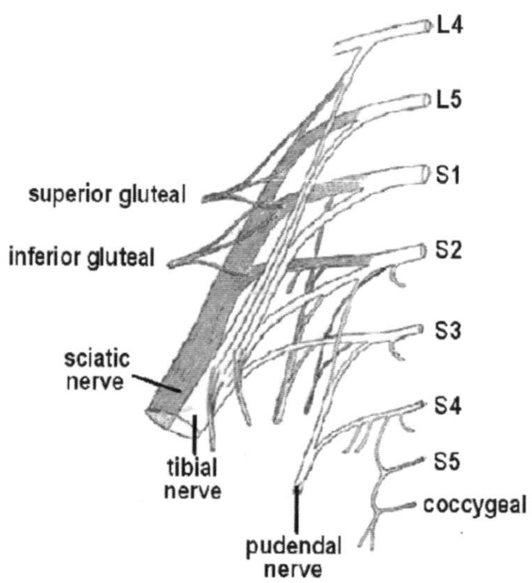

Sympathetic Splanchnic Nerves

With the exception of the pelvic splanchnic nerves, the splanchnic (visceral) nerves are all sympathetic fibers. The postsynaptic cardiopulmonary fibers originate in the cervical and upper thoracic ganglia to innervate the thoracic cavity. The thoracic splanchnic nerves are presynaptic nerves that innervate the abdominal viscera. The greater splanchnic nerve arises from T5 through T9 or T10; its fibers synapse in the celiac ganglion and act upon the foregut enteric nervous system (ENS). The lesser splanchnic nerves arise from T9 or T10 through T11 or T12; their fibers synapse in the superior mesenteric ganglia or aorticorenal ganglion, where they modulate the midgut ENS. The least splanchnic nerve arises from T11–L2 or T12, and synapses in the renal ganglia to innervate the kidneys, the spermatic plexus, and the inferior vena cava. The lumbar splanchnic nerves are presynaptic fibers from L1 and L2 that synapse in the inferior mesenteric ganglia of the intermesenteric plexus and the hypogastric plexus. The sacral splanchnic nerves are presynaptic fibers from the sacrum that synapse in the inferior hypogastric plexus and the pelvic visceral ganglia.

Parasympathetic Nerves

The parasympathetic nerves arise from cranial nerves 3, 7, 9, and 10 and the lateral gray horns of the sacral spine (S2–S4). Their long preganglionic fibers extend from the CNS to ganglia close to or embedded within their target organs. Their postganglionic fibers are correspondingly short in contrast to the sympathetic fibers. Cranial nerves 3 to 9 innervate the organs and glands of the face and head. Fibers from the vagus nerve (cranial nerve 10) run to the organs of the thoracic and abdominal cavities. The sacral parasympathetic nerves, known as the pelvic splanchnic nerves, innervate the descending and sigmoid colon, the inferior hypogastric plexus, and the pelvic viscera.

Tactile Receptors in the Skin

Mechanical and thermal stimuli are detected by nerve termini located throughout the skin and in certain internal regions such as joints. The somae of these afferent somatic fibers are located in the dorsal root ganglia, and their axons synapse with interneurons in the dorsal horn of the spinal cord. Nociceptors are triggered once a minimum threshold stimulus is received. Four types of tactile receptors are found in the skin: Pacinian corpuscles, Meissner's corpuscles, Merkel discs, and Ruffini nerve endings. Deep pressure and vibration on the skin surface are detected by Pacinian corpuscles. Light pressure is picked up by Merkel discs, which are involved in shape and texture discrimination. Meissner's corpuscles are also sensitive to light touch as well as low frequency vibrations. Ruffini nerve endings detect both temperature and the stretching of skin, and are involved in the kinesthetic control of finger movement and the delicate manipulation of objects. Pain and other noxious temperature and chemical stimuli are detected by superficial and deeper nociceptors with free nerve endings.

Pacinian corpuscle, a Meissner's corpuscle, and Ruffini's nerve endings:

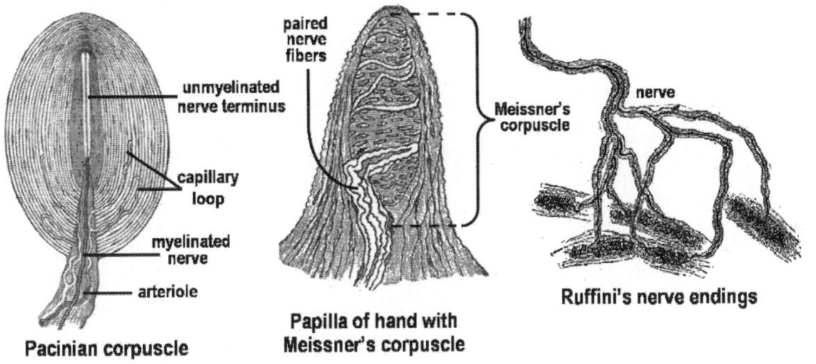

Pathways of Tactile Signals to the Brain

Afferent neurons bringing signals from the lower body about touch, pressure, and vibration enter the spinal cord at T7 or below; those coming in from the upper body enter at T6 and above. Both synapse in the dorsal horn (in the gracile fasciculus and the cuneate fasciculus, respectively) with ascending fibers, which carry the signals to the brainstem. These signals are sent to the ipsilateral thalamus via this medial lemniscal system. Pain and temperature messages are routed to the contralateral thalamus (and then to the higher cortex) via the anterolateral system. Proprioceptive signals from muscle spindles and Golgi tendon organs about the position of the limbs and joints are sent to the ipsilateral cerebellum via the spinocerebellar tract.

Cross section of the spinal cord:

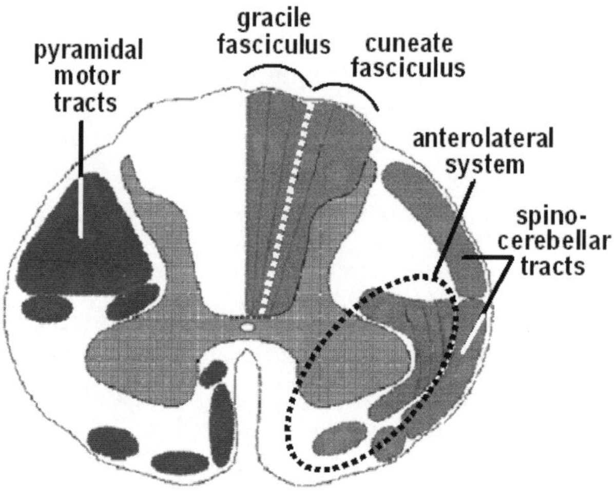

Embryonic Origin of the Peripheral Nervous System

The peripheral nervous system is derived largely from migratory neural crest cells. This includes the dorsal root ganglia and afferent sensory neurons of the spinal nerves, the Schwann cells of all peripheral nerves, the satellite glial cells of the sensory and autonomic ganglia, the sympathetic and parasympathetic postganglionic fibers, and the visceral neural plexus of the various distal tissues and organs. Migratory neural crest cells also differentiate into melanocyte stem cells, which give rise to Merkel discs and many other types of cells. Efferent motor neurons develop from the ventral roots that emerge from the spinal cord.

Olfaction

Humans have between 40 and 50 million bipolar olfactory receptor neurons (ORNs) capable of detecting 10,000 or more distinct odors. Tiny cilia extend from the dendrites of each ORN into the mucus-covered olfactory epithelium lining the nasal cavity. The ORN axons penetrate perforations in the cribriform plate of the ethmoid bone to synapse with the dendrites of mitral cells inside spherical glomeruli located just inside the olfactory bulb. The mitral cells carry the olfactory signals via the lateral olfactory tract to five major regions of the cerebral cortex: the anterior olfactory nucleus, the olfactory tubercle, the piriform cortex, the entorhinal cortex, and the amygdala. The piriform cortex also sends signals to the thalamus, the hypothalamus, the hippocampus, and other portions of the limbic system. For this reason, odors often evoke powerful emotional responses.

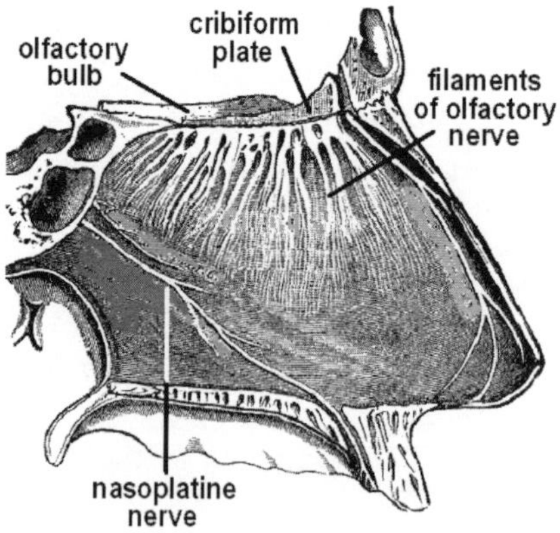

Relationships among the olfactory receptor nerves, the olfactory epithelium, the mitral cells, the glomeruli, and the olfactory bulb:

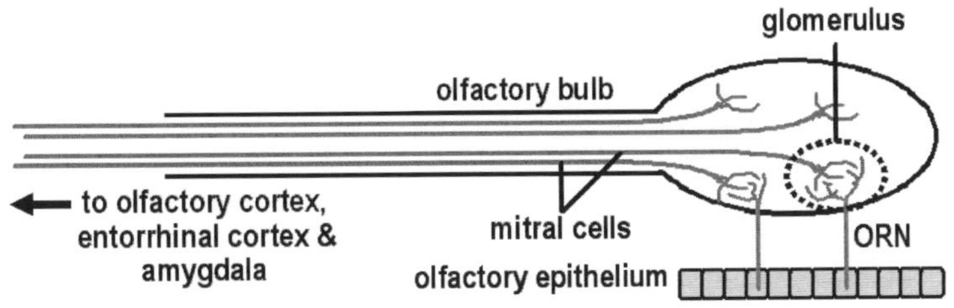

HUMAN EYE

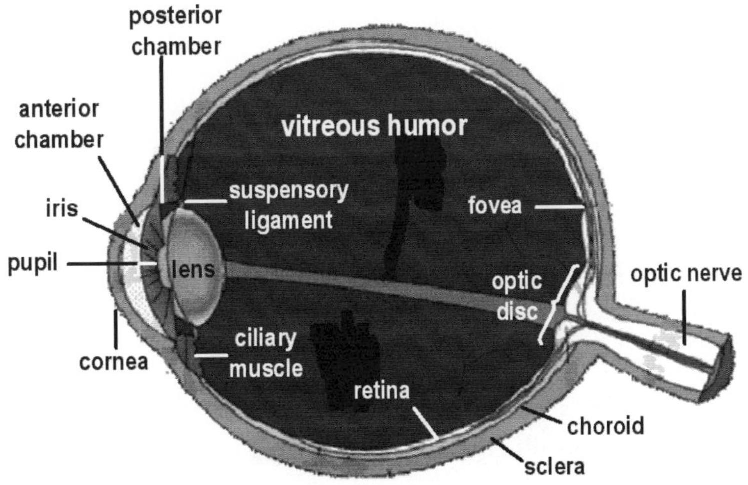

HUMAN RETINA

The pigmented layer of the retina lies against the sclera; the innermost layer consists of neurons from the optic tract, which abut the hyaloid membrane of the vitreous humor. Light passes through the pupil, travels through the vitreous humor, and passes through the transparent nerve layer to reach the photoreceptive rods and cones in the rear. Rhodopsin consists of a protein (opsin) reversibly bonded to retinal, an aldehyde of vitamin A. Absorption of a photon isomerizes 11-*cis*-retinal to all-*trans*-retinal. This initiates a nervous impulse back to the nerves via the horizontal cells, the bipolar cells, and the amacrine cells, which then travels to the optic nerves. Rhodopsin is found in the rods, and functions in dim light. Four other photopsins occur in the cones, and play a vital role in color vision and visual acuity.

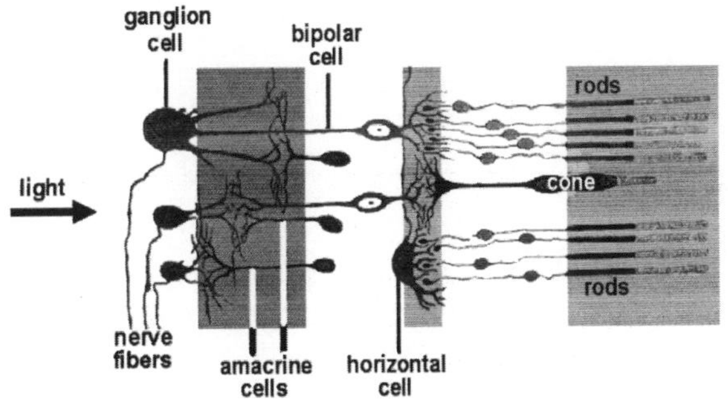

Pathways taken by signals from the retinae to the visual cortex: In primates, images of objects in the left visual field will strike the nasal part of the left retina and the temporal part of the retina. They will then be sent along the right optic tract to the right lateral geniculate in the thalamus, and then to the visual cortex. The situation is reversed for objects in the right visual field. Images from the right will impinge upon the temporal region of the left retina and the nasal region of the right retina. From there, they will travel along the left optic tract to the left lateral geniculate nucleus, and then to the visual cortex. The image shows the pathway of signals from the left visual field. To enable binocular vision, information from the two visual fields is kept separate until it reaches the visual cortex.

Embryogenesis of the Eye

The mammalian eye is a direct outgrowth of the diencephalon, the optic vesicles, which emerge by week three. As such, the optic nerve and the retina are part of the central nervous system, and the optic nerve is properly termed the optic tract. It is enclosed within the meninges, and the myelin sheathing its fibers is produced by oligodendrocytes. When the optic vesicles contact the overlying ectoderm, it induces the epithelium to thicken and form the lens placode. As the lens differentiates, it invaginates, separates from the epithelium, and induces the epidermis to develop into the cornea and the optic vesicle to differentiate into the optic cup. The two layers of the optic cup in turn develop into an inner retina and an outer pigmented retinal layer. Nearby mesenchymal cells induce the development of the optic nerve, and also develop into the iris, the ciliary body, the sclera, and the blood vessels of the eye.

Developmental Stages of the Optic Cup and the Optic Tract

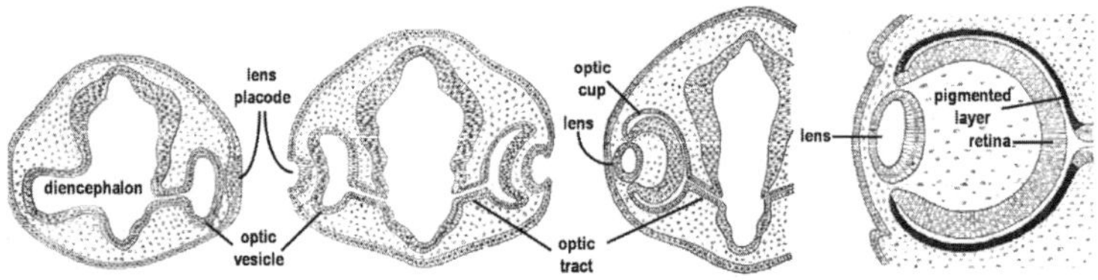

Human Ear

The outer ear includes the pinna, the ear canal, and the tympanic membrane. The middle ear includes the three ossicles—the malleus, the incus, and the stapes—and the opening of the Eustachian tube. The inner ear is embedded in a bony labyrinth within the temporal bone. It comprises the membranous labyrinth, and consists of the vestibule, the semicircular canals, and the cochlea. The membranous labyrinth is filled with potassium-rich fluid called endolymph. Between it and the hard bony labyrinth is a fluid called perilymph. The vestibule and semicircular canals have functions related to the detection of position orientation, balance, and motion. Within the vestibule, two otolith organs sense gravity and linear acceleration. Three perpendicularly arranged, semicircular canals detect rotational motion along the pitch, roll, and yaw axes. This information is transmitted to the brain by the vestibular nerve. Sound waves gathered by the pinna and carried through the ear canal cause the tympanic membrane to vibrate. These vibrations are transmitted by the endolymph to the cochlea, where they initiate nerve signals in the cochlear nerve.

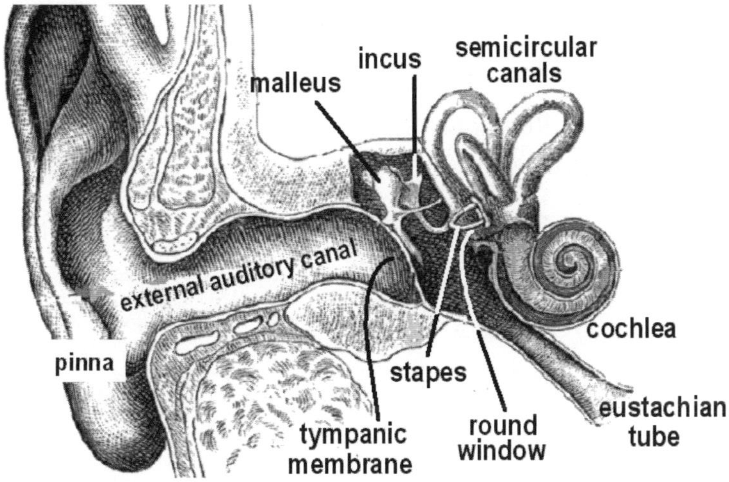

DETECTION OF SOUND IN INNER EAR

The outer and middle ear in humans and terrestrial mammals are filled with air. The Eustachian tube connects the middle ear to the nasopharynx. Aerial sound waves cause the tympanic membrane to vibrate. These vibrations are transmitted through the middle ear via the three ear ossicles to the footplate of the stapes. This initiates corresponding vibrations in the endolymph, filling the three canals inside the coiled, snail-like cochlea: the scala vestibuli, the scala media, and the scala tympani. Movements of the fluid in the scala media stimulate the tectorial membrane and the cilia on hair cells in the organ of Corti. These, in turn, initiate nervous impulses, which are carried in the cochlear nerve (the auditory portion of the eighth cranial nerve) to the brain. The location of the hair cells along the cochlea that are stimulated by the sound vibration frequencies determines the pitch of the sound perceived by the brain.

COCHLEA AND ORGAN OF CORTI

Structures of the cochlea and the organ of Corti:

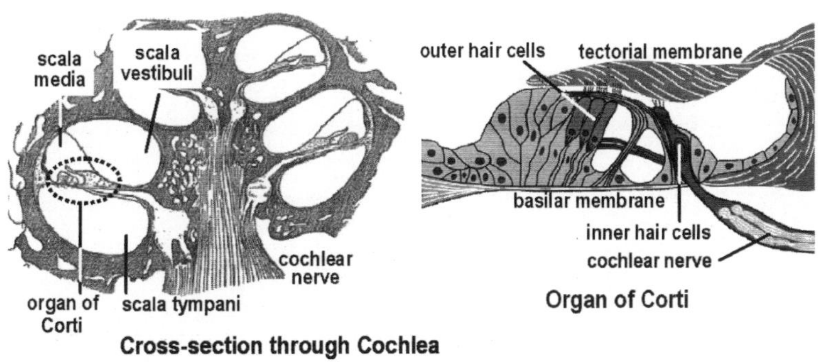

EMBRYOGENESIS OF THE MIDDLE AND INNER EAR ELEMENTS

The three ossicles and the tympanic membrane of the middle ear are formed from portions of Meckel's cartilage, which ossifies to become the dentary bone (lower jaw). The portions that give rise to the middle ear structures later break away and migrate to lie adjacent to the inner ear. The inner ear begins developing from a pair of otic placodes during the third week of gestation. These ectodermal thickenings evaginate and move next to the rhombencephalon. They then separate from the ectoderm to become the fluid-filled otic vesicles. These then develop into the utricle and saccule (the vestibular organs), the three semicircular canals, and the vestibulocochlear ganglion complex. The malleus, the incus, the stapes, and the tympanic membrane are homologous with the articular, the quadrate, the periarticular, and the angular of the reptilian jaw. The stapes is derived from the reptilian columella, which evolved earlier from the hyomandibular, one of the gill arches in early vertebrates.

Embryonic Formation of the Inner Ear

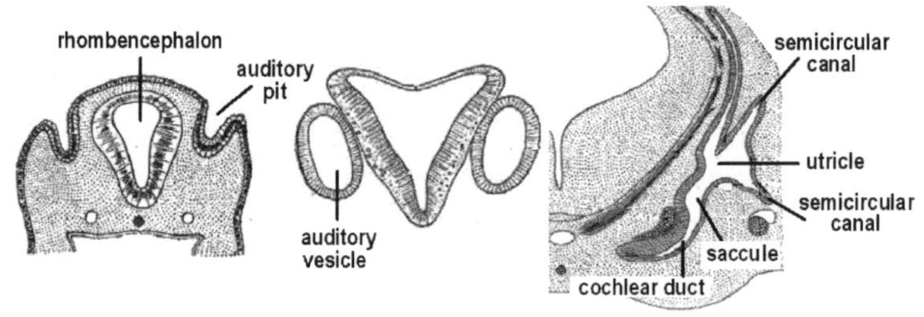

Gustation

The top of the human tongue has 2,000 to 8,000 taste buds, each enclosed within a raised papilla with a taste pore opening to the oral cavity. Taste receptors are also located in the palate, the larynx, and the upper esophagus. Food and other molecules dissolved in the saliva enter the taste pores, where they are detected by specialized receptor cells. When activated, these receptors initiate action potentials that are conveyed to the brain via the 7th (facial), 9th (glossopharyngeal), and 10th (vagus) cranial nerves. The major components of taste perception are salty, sour, bitter, sweet, and *umami*—an untranslatable Japanese term describing the taste of glutamates and nucleotides. The *umami* taste along with olfaction balance and enhance all the flavors in a meal and contribute to its overall "palatability." The erroneous idea that different flavors are confined to different regions of the tongue is still widely taught using a "tongue map" visual. However, all parts of the tongue can taste every flavor, even though certain regions are more sensitive to specific flavors than others.

Physiology

Lateralization of the Brain

The brain is split into two cerebral hemispheres that are essentially mirror images of each other. Each hemisphere connects primarily with the opposite side of the body, and the two cerebral hemispheres are connected via the corpus callosum just above the level of the paired thalami. Minor connections also exist, such as the anterior commissure and the intermediate mass. Efferent connections from the brain and afferent connections from the body cross to the opposite side in the brainstem. Autonomic functions are controlled by the lower half of the brainstem (medulla oblongata). Certain language functions and logical reasoning are lateralized in the left hemisphere in nearly 90 percent of right-handed individuals, but these functions occur in the right brain in only half of left-handed persons.

Limbic System

The limbic system, or old mammalian brain, has functions related to emotion, behavior, long-term memory, and smell. It consists of structures of the lower cortex as well as the diencephalon, and also includes portions of the thalamus (the relay station of the brain), the septum pellucidum, the hippocampus, the amygdala, the fornix, and the mammillary bodies. It also includes the parahippocampal, the cingulate, the dentate gyri, the nucleus accumbens, and other regions of the lower cortex.

Basal Ganglia

The basal ganglia include several interconnected nuclei of diverse origin at the base of the forebrain that connect with the cerebral cortex, the thalamus, and other regions of the brain. They include, among other structures, the striatum (the caudate nucleus and the putamen), the globus pallidus, the amygdala, the substantia nigra, and the ventral tegmental area in the midbrain. These structures function together in emotional behavior, sexuality, the experience of and reactions to fear and rage, and the conversion of short-term memory to long-term memory.

Subdivisions of the Nervous System

The central nervous system (CNS) consists of the brain and the spinal cord. The peripheral nervous system (PNS) includes the ganglia and nerves lying outside the CNS. It connects the limbs, trunk, and viscera to the CNS. Though the cranial nerves originate in the brain, their axons extend well into the periphery, and they are considered part of the PNS. The PNS, in turn, is divided into the somatic nervous system that innervates the skeletal muscles and is under voluntary control, and the autonomic nervous system (ANS), which innervates the viscera and glands of the body and is largely under involuntary control.

Resting Potential in Nervous Tissue

Neurons, like muscle cells, are enclosed in an excitable plasma membrane (the neurilemma). (The neurilemma is only slightly permeable to Na^+, but it is highly permeable to K^+. These ions tend to leak down their concentration gradient from the cytosol to the cell exterior.) A sodium-potassium-dependent ATPase (the "sodium potassium pump") driven by ATP establishes a resting potential of about $^-70$ millivolts across the membrane. The sodium potassium pump transports 2 K^+ inside the membrane and 3 Na^+ to the outside of the membrane at the cost of 1 ATP molecule. This sets up a net surfeit of positive ions (Na^+ and K^+) outside the membrane relative to the inside. The inside of the membrane is thus some 70 mV less positive than the outside. The transmission of a nervous impulse involves the depolarization of the resting potential. This is accomplished by opening ionic channels that specifically permit Na^+ to flow down its concentration gradient from the outside of the cell to the inside.

Neuron

The basic structural and functional unit of the nervous system is the nerve cell, or neuron. A series of afferent fibers called dendrites are attached to the soma, or cell body, which contains a nucleus and all the necessary cellular organelles and machinery. At the base of the soma is a swelling known as the axon hillock, and beyond that stretches an efferent fiber (axon) of varying length. At the axon terminal are a series of short fibers capped by slight swellings called terminal buttons. This is followed by a small gap, the synaptic cleft (or simply the synapse), beyond which lie the dendrites and/or cell body of the next neuron in the series. The axons of many (but certainly not all) neurons are enclosed in a series of electrochemically insulating myelin sheaths, with the bare axon exposed only at narrow caps called nodes of Ranvier.

Basic neuron:

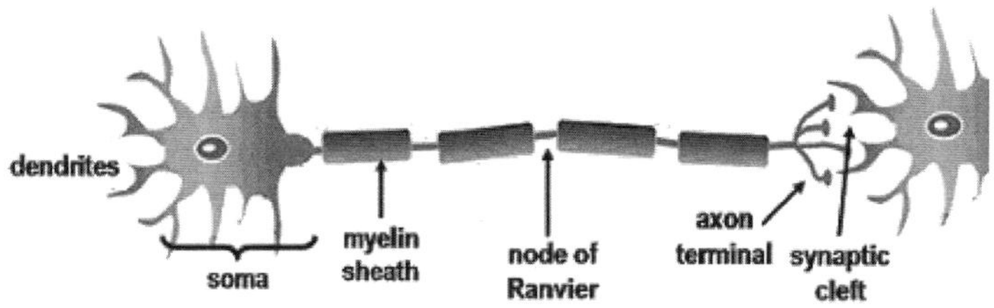

Graded Potential

A graded potential is a graduated depolarization, the intensity of which varies according to the strength of the incoming stimulus. It occurs on the dendrites and the soma, and the response attenuates over both space and time. In response to neurotransmitter substances (see below), Na^+ ions flow down chemically gated channels on the postsynaptic membrane to effect this depolarization. Graded potentials can be excitatory (as in this case) or inhibitory, in which Cl^- ions enter the neuron through chloride channels and hyperpolarize the membrane by increasing the internal sum of minus charges. The resting potential is thus increased, requiring a greater sum of excitatory potentials to generate an action potential.

Action Potential

An action potential is an all-or-nothing, short-acting *polarity reversal* that occurs when the sum total of all excitatory and inhibitory graded potentials reaches the axon hillock at a threshold intensity, usually about +40 to +55 mV. When this happens, adjacent voltage-gated channels on the axon suddenly open wide, and Na^+ ions rush inside the membrane and completely reverse the resting potential. It is now more positive inside the membrane than outside; the resting potential of -70 mV has been reversed to between +40 and +100 mV. This is immediately followed by the opening of K^+ channels, allowing K^+ to exit the neuron and reestablish the original polarity. However, the ion species are reversed. This is the absolute refractory period, during which the neuron cannot fire again. Eventually, the sodium potassium pump kicks in again and gradually restores the original resting potential, with the Na^+ and K^+ ions in their correct locations. The neuron is again ready to fire.

When the action potential sweeps into the axon terminal, it causes Ca^{2+} channels to open. The influx of Ca^{2+} causes synaptic vesicles in the terminal buttons laden with one or more specific neurotransmitters to fuse with the presynaptic membrane and release its contents through exocytosis. Common excitatory neurotransmitters include acetylcholine (ACh) and norepinephrine (NE) in the peripheral and autonomic nervous systems. Glutamate predominates in the central nervous system (CNS). Inhibitory neurotransmitters in the CNS include dopamine, 5-hydroxytryptamine (serotonin), gamma-aminobutyric acid (GABA), and glycine (found in the spinal cord, the brainstem, and the retina). The neurotransmitter molecules diffuse across the synaptic gap and bind to specific receptors on the postsynaptic membrane (the neurilemma enclosing the dendrite or soma on the other side of the gap). These receptors are associated with chemically-gated ion channels that initiate postsynaptic graded potentials.

Saltatory Nerve Conduction

Action potentials trigger new action potentials on adjacent sections of the axon, which propagate without attenuation. In the case of myelinated neurons such as those that predominate in the somatic nervous system, the action potential only occurs at the nodes of Ranvier, and the nervous impulse moves by jumping from node to node. This bypasses most of the length of the axon (which may be a meter or more long). This saltatory conduction enables extremely rapid transmission of the nervous impulse, which occurs in a reflex arc.

Subdivisions of the Autonomic Nervous System

The ANS is divided into the sympathetic nervous system and the parasympathetic nervous system, which are responsible for "flight-or-fight" responses to real and perceived threats and restoration to normal baseline status, respectively. The sympathetic nerves arise from the thoracic and lumbar vertebrae, and release acetylcholine (Ach) from the short, preganglionic fibers and norepinephrine (NE) from the postganglionic fibers. These activate nicotinic receptors on the postganglionic fibers and adrenergic receptors on the target cells, respectively. The craniosacral parasympathetic nerves arise from the cranial nerves 3, 7, 9, and 10 and the sacral nerves S2–S4. They release Ach from both the long preganglionic fibers and short postganglionic fibers. The preganglionic fibers activate nicotinic receptors; the postganglionic fibers activate muscarinic receptors on the target cells. A third component of the ANS is the enteric nervous system (ENS), a largely autonomous system that innervates the gut and releases serotonin as a major neurotransmitter. It operates largely independently of the CNS to control peristalsis and the secretion of digestive enzymes.

Simple Reflex Arc

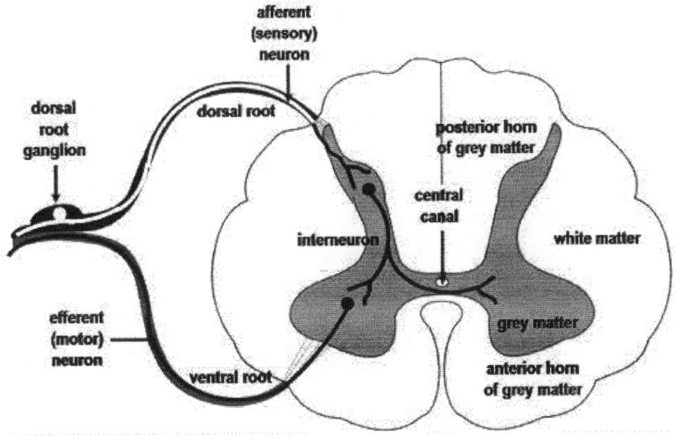

Sagittal Section of the Brain

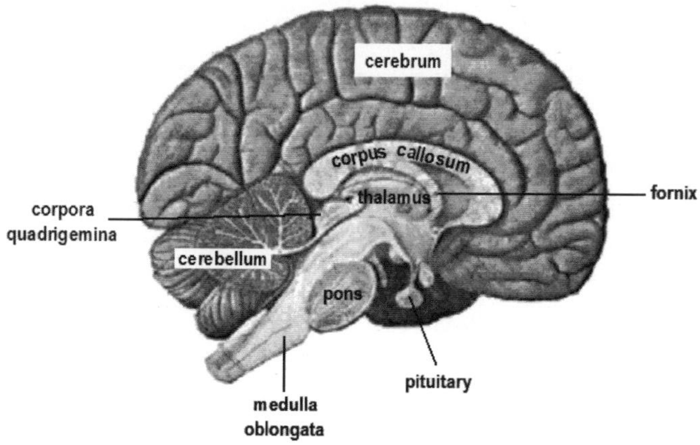

Cerebral Cortex

Each cerebral hemisphere is divided into a frontal lobe, a parietal lobe, a temporal lobe, and an occipital lobe. The frontal lobe is involved with reasoning, movement, logic, problem solving, and abstract thinking. The parietal lobe integrates sensory input, and is involved in spatial orientation and navigation. The temporal lobe receives auditory input and functions in semantics; it includes the hippocampus, and is also involved in memory. The occipital lobe is associated with vision.

Diencephalon

The diencephalon of the brain is comprised of the paired thalami, the epithalamus, and the hypothalamus, which enclose the third ventricle. The thalamus is the relay center of the brain that routes afferent signals from the spinal cord and efferent signals from the cerebral cortex to their proper destinations. The epithalamus contains the pineal gland and the corpora quadrigemina (responsible for relaying visual and auditory signals), as well as the choroid plexus. The hypothalamus has functions related to temperature regulation, thirst, satiety, and electrolyte balance. It also plays a role in regulating other autonomic functions, and works together with the pituitary gland as a neuroendocrine system.

Cerebellum

The cerebellum is located below the occipital lobes and dorsal to the brainstem. It receives afferent signals from the muscles, joints, and semicircular canals of the inner ear, and it sends efferent messages to the reticular formation (involved in arousal, sleep, consciousness, pain modulation, and habituation), the vestibular nucleus, and the thalamus. It is involved in the coordination of movement, balance, and skilled voluntary motor activity, including speech and writing.

Skeletal Muscle

Each skeletal muscle is wrapped in a connective tissue sheath (epimysium) containing many individual muscles cells (myofibers). These are grouped in discrete bundles (fascicles), each of which is wrapped in a connective tissue sheath (perimysium). Each myofiber in turn is wrapped in connective tissue (the endomysium), and contains long, rod-like groups of contractile myofibrils. These connective tissue sheaths are continuous with each other and with the tendons that attach the muscle to the bones. The contractile unit is the sarcomere, which consists of groups of thick myosin filaments surrounded by thin (actin) filaments and bounded at both ends by a Z disc. The thick filaments are attached to each Z disc by elastic (titin) filaments. Each muscle is innervated by one nerve, an artery, and several veins that enter/exit near the belly and branch throughout the connective tissue sheaths. Like all cell plasma membranes, the sarcolemma of a muscle cell has a resting potential.

Anatomic features of a skeletal muscle:

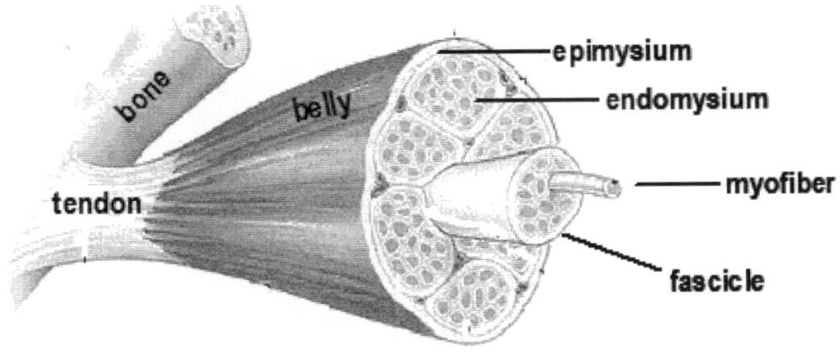

SARCOMERE

Structure of a sarcomere

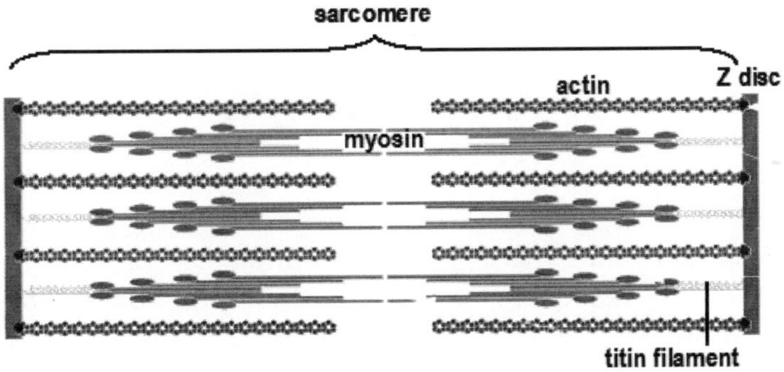

MUSCLE CONTRACTION

An incoming action potential releases ACh at the muscle cell motor end plate and generates an action potential. This action potential spreads throughout the sarcolemma down through T tubules, and then throughout an elaborate sarcoplasmic reticulum (SR) that surrounds each myofibril. Ca^{2+} is released from the terminal cisternae of the SR, which binds to troponin molecules attached to tropomyosin on the surface of the actin filaments. This troponin changes shape and removes the blocking action of tropomyosin, which exposes the actin's active sites. This allows the heads of the myosin filaments to alternately bind and detach from the actin. This process results in the release of ADP and Pi, causing the cocked myosin heads to swivel, which pulls the actin filaments toward the centerline of the sarcomere. A new ATP molecule then binds to the myosin heads, causing them to detach from the actin and become cocked and ready to repeat the cycle.

SKELETAL, CARDIAC, AND SMOOTH MUSCLE

Skeletal (voluntary) muscle is a syncytium of multinucleated, longitudinal, striated muscles cells, each of which is innervated by a motor nerve. An efferent nervous impulse is needed to initiate muscle cell contraction. In contrast, involuntary, striated cardiac muscle cells contain one, two, or four nuclei at most, and are often branched. Each cardiomyocyte is connected to its neighbors by intercalated discs, which enables synchronized contraction of heart muscle tissue. Smooth muscle consists of involuntary, nonstriated, mononucleated cells found in the walls of blood and lymphatic vessels, the bladder, the reproductive tracts of both sexes, the gut, the respiratory tract, the dermis, and the iris and lens of the eye.

Circulation of Blood Through the Heart

Deoxygenated blood enters the right atrium (3) via the superior (1) and inferior (2) *venae cavae*, and passes into the right ventricle (4) via the tricuspid valve. From there, it is pumped out through the pulmonary artery (5, 6) to the lungs, where oxygenation takes place. The freshly oxygenated blood is carried back to the heart via the pulmonary veins (7), and enters the left atrium (8). Then, it passes through the bicuspid (mitral) valve into the left ventricle (9), and is pumped out through the aorta (10) to the body.

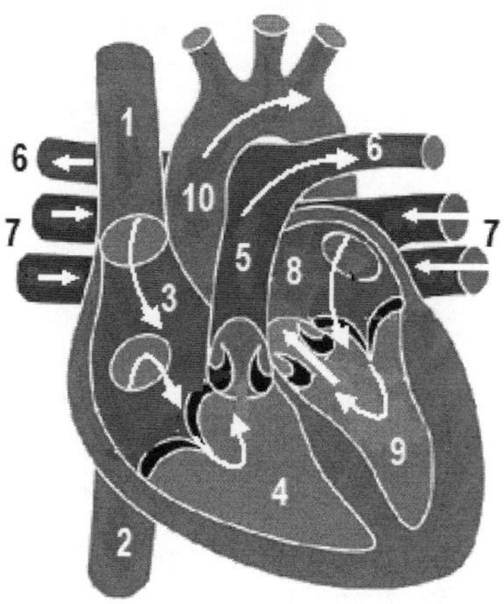

Contractions of the Heart

The sinoatrial (SA) node, or pacemaker, is a group of modified cardiac cells next to the opening of the superior vena cava that spontaneously initiates the rhythmic (60 to 100 beats per minute) contractions of the heart. Impulses from the SA node are sent to the atrioventricular (AV) node situated between the left atrium and the left ventricle. After a delay of 0.12 seconds, these impulses are then transmitted through the bundle of His (atrioventricular bundle) to the right and left branches, which innervate the right and left ventricles, respectively. The AV node can also initiate contractile impulses, but its slower rate (40 to 60 beats per minute) is normally overridden by the SA node. The spontaneous impulses of the SA node are modulated by the opposing parasympathetic and sympathetic actions of the vagus nerve and the spinal nerves (T–T4), respectively.

Electrical Stimulation of the Heart

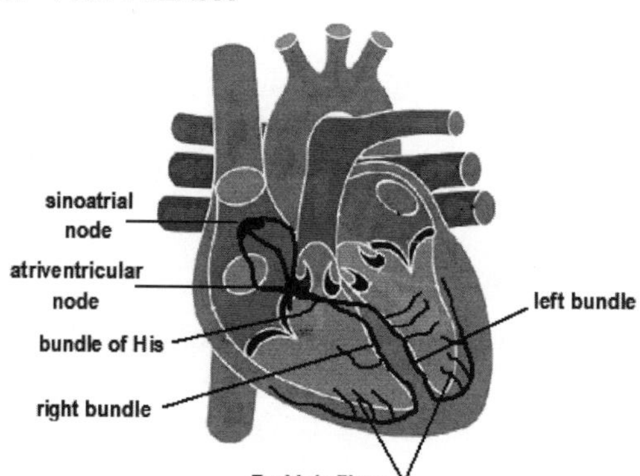

Hemodynamics

Hemodynamics deals with cardiac output and vascular resistance to blood flow through the body. Many factors influence blood flow, including CO_2 levels, blood volume and viscosity, laminar versus turbulent flow, and vascular diameter, length, and resistance. These factors are in turn affected by diet, drugs/medications, disease, exercise, and body mass. The flow of blood is generally calculated using the formula $F = \Delta P/R = P_A - P_V/R$, where F = blood flow and ΔP = the difference in pressure between two points along a blood vessel. The pressure difference in an organ is determined by calculating the difference between the arterial (P_A) and venous (P_V) pressures.

Regulation of Blood Flow

The most important factor in regulating blood flow through arteries and organs is changes in vessel diameter. Vasoconstricting and vasodilating chemicals and myogenic constriction and relaxation in response to changes in blood pressure are important local tissue regulators. Autonomic signals from the sympathetic and parasympathetic nervous systems and circulating vasoactive hormones such as epinephrine and norepinephrine, angiotensin II, vasopressin, atrial natriuretic peptide, and endothelin also play prominent roles by fine tuning vascular resistance.

Lymphatic System

Part of the overall circulatory system, the lymphatic vessels carry the lymph, a fluid derived from the interstitial fluid (which is itself derived from plasma constituents leaving the capillaries) and chyle from the intestines back to where these fluids drain into the circulating blood via one of two subclavian veins. The lymphatic system includes the lymphoid tissues and lymph nodes, the lacteals associated with the gut, and the tonsils and adenoids. It also includes the bone marrow, the thymus, and the spleen, which are organs, glands, and tissues involved in the generation of lymphocytes and white blood cells.

Lymph Capillaries and Vessels

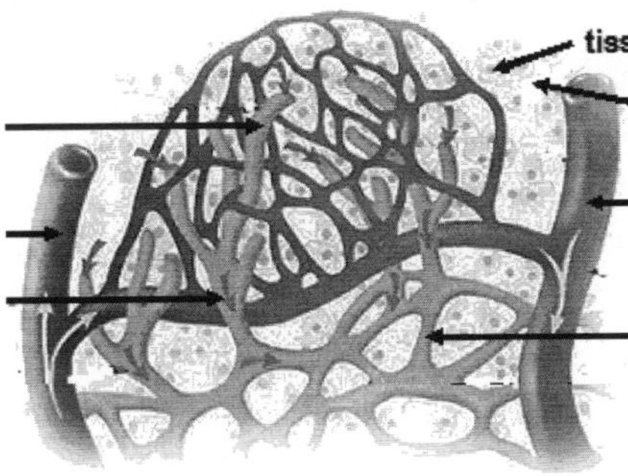

Hematology

Hematology is the study of blood (a mesodermally derived liquid connective tissue), as well as its plasma matrix and formed elements (blood cells and platelets); the blood-forming organs; and the diagnosis, etiology, prevention, and treatment of the diseases of the blood. Hematopathologists are pathologists specializing in the diagnosis of hematological diseases who often work with hematologists to arrive at diagnoses and appropriate treatment options for blood diseases.

Breathing

Breathing (ventilation) involves active inspiration and passive expiration. During inspiration, the diaphragm and intercostal muscles contract, increasing the volume of the chest cavity and reducing the air pressure inside the alveoli so that it is lower than the ambient atmospheric pressure. Air rushes into the lungs through the respiratory tract and fills the alveoli. During expiration, the diaphragm and intercostal muscles relax, and the chest cavity returns to its original volume. This increases the internal alveolar pressure, forcing the air back out.

External Respiration

External respiration involves the gaseous exchange of O_2 and CO_2 between the air in the approximately 300 million alveoli and the blood in their surrounding capillaries. Deoxygenated blood enters the lungs through the pulmonary arteries, its CO_2 is given up in exchange for O_2 in the freshly inspired air, and the freshly oxygenated blood is returned to the heart via the pulmonary veins. The approximate respective pO_2 and pCO_2 values (mm Hg) are as follows: inspired air, 149 and 0.3; alveolar air, 100 and 40; pulmonary arteries, 40 and 46; and pulmonary veins, 95 and 40. The pulmonary arterial and venous partial pressures are reversed in systemic circulation. This ensures that deoxygenated blood will exchange CO_2 for alveolar O_2, sending freshly charged oxygenated blood to the heart for distribution throughout the body.

Internal Respiration

Internal respiration is the exchange of oxygen and carbon dioxide between the arterioles and the peripheral tissues. The tissues maintain fairly constant pO_2s and pCO_2s of less than 30 mm Hg and more than 40 mm Hg, respectively. This ensures that O_2 will be taken up and CO_2 will be given off by actively metabolizing tissue cells. The relative pO_2s and pCO_2s are accordingly reversed in the returning venous flow to the heart, which is then sent to the lungs via the pulmonary arteries, where external respiration occurs.

Lung Volumes and Capacities

The average total lung capacities (TLC) at maximum inflation of an adult male and female lung are 6 liters and 4.2 liters, respectively. Other measures include the following: residual volume (RV), which is the volume of air remaining after maximal exhalation; expiratory reserve volume (ERV), which is the maximum volume that can be exhaled from the end-expiratory position; inspiratory reserve volume (IRV), which is the maximum volume that can be inhaled from the end-inspiratory level; tidal volume (TV or V_T), which is the volume moved in or out of the lungs during quiet breathing (when precisely measured, this is symbolized by VT or V_T); inspiratory capacity (IC), which is the sum of IRV and TV; inspiratory vital capacity (IVC), which is the maximum volume of air inhaled from the point of maximum expiration; vital capacity (VC), which is the difference between TLC and RV; and FEV1, which is the volume of air exhaled after one second of forced expiration.

Factors That Control Respiration Rate

Blood pH is detected by receptors in the medulla oblongata, and levels of O_2 and CO_2 are measured by the carotid and aortic bodies in the carotid arteries and the aorta, respectively. Respiration rate is controlled by the inspiratory and expiratory centers in the medulla oblongata and the pneumotaxic (inhibits inspiration) and apneustic (stimulates inspiration) centers in the pons. As CO_2 levels increase with metabolic rate (under exertion, for example), the bicarbonate buffering equation is shifted in favor of increasing proton buildup: $CO_2 + H_2O \leftrightarrow H_2CO_3 \leftrightarrow HCO_3^- + H^+$, thus lowering the blood pH.

How Oxygen Is Carried in the Blood

At rest, the body needs about 250 mL/min of O_2. More than 98 percent of the O_2 is combined with hemoglobin (Hb) in the red blood cells to form oxyhemoglobin, while less than two percent is dissolved in the plasma. Each Hb tetramer can carry up to four O_2 molecules. The binding of O_2 to Hb depends on the serum pCO_2 and the binding affinity between Hb and O_2. Hb saturation is determined by the partial pressure of oxygen. At high pO_2s, Hb has a high affinity for O_2. Hb may be 98 percent saturated in the lungs, where the pO_2 is around 100 mm Hg. Tissue pO_2s are much lower (about 40 mm Hg). Here, Hb has a much lower oxygen binding affinity, and releases some of its O_2

to the tissues. It still remains 75 percent saturated, however. Actively contracting muscle has a pO_2 of about 20 mm Hg. Here, Hb is only 35 percent saturated. Decreasing pH and increasing temperature and pCO2 (during exercise, for instance) also lower the binding affinity of Hb for O_2.

How Carbon Dioxide Is Carried in the Blood

About 7 to 10 percent of the CO_2 released from the tissues is dissolved in the blood. Where the pCO_2 is low (as in the alveoli), dissolved CO_2 comes out of solution and is exhaled. Most of the CO_2 is carried in the blood as HCO_3^- to prevent the buildup of H^+ and the lowering of serum pH.

Nephron

The nephron is the functional unit of the kidney. It filters wastes from the blood, and regulates electrolyte and other ion levels. It also regulates the pH, volume, and pressure of the blood. It in turn is regulated by the hypothalamic-pituitary-adrenal axis. Each nephron consists of a renal corpuscle. Each corpuscle consists of a Bowman's capsule enclosing the glomerulus, as well as a capillary knot fed by an afferent vessel and drained by an efferent vessel. The renal corpuscle connects with the renal tubule, which consists of (1) the proximal convoluted tubule, (2) the deep, U-shaped loop of Henle with a descending and ascending limb, and (3) the distal convoluted tubule. The nephron drains into the collecting tubule, and from there into the collecting duct, which drains the urine via the ureter into the bladder.

Basic Function

Proteins under 30 kDa and smaller molecules like water, NaCl, glucose, amino acids, and urea are readily filtered from the glomerular blood to produce a filtrate very similar to blood plasma. This filtrate passes into the Bowman's space, and then into (1) the proximal convoluted tubule, (2) the loop of Henle, (3) the distal convoluted tubule, and (4) the collecting tubules and ducts (here it exists as the urine). Solutes and water are reabsorbed into the renal interstitium from the tubular filtrate, and then back into the blood. The descending limb of the loop is highly permeable to water and fairly permeable to salt, which pass freely into the hypertonic interstitium through osmosis. The ascending limb is impermeable to water, while Na^+ is actively pumped out via a $Na^+/K^+/2Cl^-$ symporter to produce the interstitial hypertonic state that drives the loop's countercurrent exchange. This all results in a dilute filtrate that enters the distal convoluted tubule, where small amounts of sodium and chloride are reabsorbed via a Na^+/Cl^- symporter.

Structure and function of a nephron:

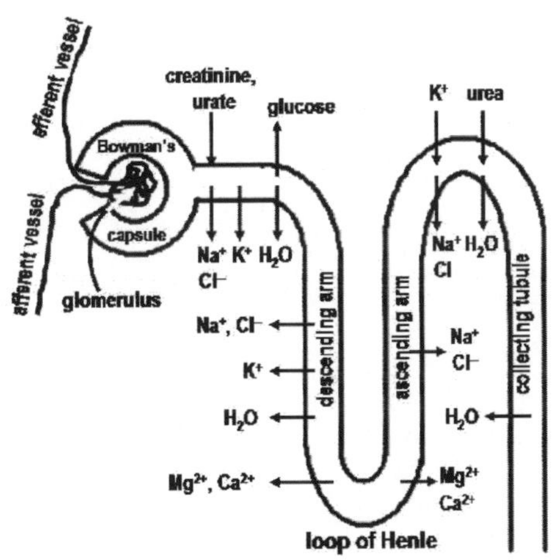

Control of Micturition

Micturition (urination) is controlled by interactions among the central, autonomic, and somatic nervous systems, as well the endocrine system. Essentially a spinobulbospinal reflex, micturition is both facilitated and suppressed by the pontine micturition center in coordination with input from periaqueductal grey matter and the medial frontal cortex. It is thus under voluntary control in healthy individuals. The detrusor muscle of the bladder is innervated by lumbar sympathetic fibers and sacral parasympathetic fibers. Vasopressin, or antidiuretic hormone (ADH), is produced by the supraoptic and paraventricular nuclei in the hypothalamus and carried via the hypophyseal portal system to the neurohypophysis (posterior pituitary gland), where it is stored. When released in response to appropriate afferent signals (e.g., increased plasma osmolality), it is released into the blood and travels to the kidneys, where it increases the water permeability of the collecting duct. This allows for the resorption of water and inhibits the production of urine.

Role of Kidneys in Maintaining Acid-Base Homeostasis

The kidneys function in pH homeostasis primarily by resorbing HCO_3^- from and excreting H^+ into the urine. Of the approximately 4500 millimoles of bicarbonate ion filtered into the urine daily, just 2 millimoles are ultimately excreted. The rest is resorbed from the proximal tubule (70 to 80 percent), the loop of Henle (10 to 20 percent), and the distal tubule and collecting ducts (5 to 10 percent). Both the proximal and distal renal tubules secrete H^+ into the urine by H-ATPase in a one-to-one exchange for the transport of Na^+ into the interstitium. Additionally, for each H^+ and Na^+ exchanged, an HCO_3^- is resorbed from the urine. Some 50 millimoles of H^+ [primarily as ammonium (NH_4^+) and weak acids like $H_2PO_4^-$] are excreted by the kidneys each day.

Digestion

Digestion involves the physical (mechanical) and chemical breakdown of food into smaller particles that can be readily absorbed by the bloodstream. It begins in the mouth with mastication and the chemical breakdown of starches by amylases in the saliva. The bolus of food then moves by peristalsis down the esophagus and into the stomach through the esophageal sphincter, where hydrochloric acid and proteases secreted by the stomach chemically break down the food into even smaller chunks. This process is aided by the mechanical churning action of the muscular stomach. After a couple of hours or so, the highly acidic chyme enters the duodenum through the pyloric sphincter. Once in the duodenum, the acidic chyme is neutralized by HCO_3^- in the pancreatic fluid, which also contains trypsinogen, chymotrypsinogen, and carboxypeptidase. These are protease zymogens which, when activated, break down peptides into their constituent amino acids, pancreatic lipase (which hydrolyzes triglycerides into monoglycerides and free fatty acids), and amylases.

Main Processes in the Small Intestine

The small intestine is divided into the duodenum, the jejunum, and the ileum. These structures are listed according to the path food takes as it is digested. Food enters the duodenum first, and then travels through the jejunum to the ileum. Most chemical digestion occurs in the short (28 to 35 cm) duodenum. Acidic chyme entering through the pylorus stimulates duodenal cells to release secretin and cholecystokinin. These hormones stimulate the release of bile from the gall bladder and the release of HCO_3^-, trypsin and chymotrypsin, lipase, and amylase from the pancreas. These released substances emulsify fats, neutralize chyme acidity, and help complete the chemical digestion of proteins, fats, and carbohydrates. The peptide fragments produced by protein breakdown are reduced to free amino acids by pancreatic carboxypeptidase and intestinal aminopeptidase. Amino acids and carbohydrates are taken up by the capillaries in the intestinal villi and lipids by specialized lymphatic vessels called lacteals. Undigested material is passed into the large intestine, where salts and water are resorbed, before being eliminated in the feces.

Main Functions of the Large Intestine

The undigested remains of food are compacted and slowly passed through the large intestine, where water, salts, and essential vitamins such as K1 (phylloquinone) and K2 (menaquinone-2) produced by the gut microflora are absorbed. Vitamin B12 is also produced by gut bacteria, but is not absorbed through the colon. Undigested food residues pass through the small intestine in two hours or less, but remain in the colon for 16 hours or longer before they are finally eliminated in the feces.

Digestive Functions

Digestion is jointly controlled by the central, autonomic, and enteric nervous systems and the endocrine system. Food entering the stomach raises the pH of the stomach and stimulates gastric stretch receptors, which in turn cause the parasympathetic release of acetylcholine by the myenteric nerve plexus and the vagus nerve. This stimulates the secretion of histamine and gastrin by the stomach. These three chemicals stimulate the release of HCl, pepsinogen, and mucus; increase gastric peristalsis; and relax the pyloric sphincter. Amino acids and partially digested fats entering the small intestine stimulate enteric neural and hormonal signals that delay gastric emptying to prevent overloading the duodenum with more chyme than it can handle. Enteric reflex circuits regulate the peristaltic contractions of the digestive tract, the exact nature of which depend on the nature of the food ingested. Gastric processing and emptying occurs roughly one to two hours after eating a meal. The passage of food through the small and large intestines typically takes three to four hours and one to two days, respectively.

Sex Hormones

The sex hormones produced by the adrenal cortex are mainly male prohormones (androgens). Small amounts of female hormones (estrogen and progestins) are also produced. Sex hormones induce the development of secondary sex characteristics at puberty. Stimulated by ACTH from the adenohypophysis, the adrenal cortex secretes 5-dehydroepiandrosterone (DHEA) from progesterone, which is derived from cholesterol. DHEA is carried to the gonads, where it is converted in several steps into testosterone in males. It is converted either directly or secondarily via testosterone into estrogens in females. At the onset of puberty, gonadotropin-releasing hormone secreted by the hypothalamus stimulates the adenohypophysis to release follicle-stimulating hormone (FSH) and luteinizing hormone (LH). FSH and LH jointly stimulate the release of estradiol and progesterone from the ovaries and testosterone from the testes, which produce ovulation in females and spermatogenesis in males, respectively.

The sex steroids play important roles in sexual development and maturation, the sex drive, and anabolism (the synthesis of complex molecules from smaller ones). Anabolic processes are necessary for the growth and differentiation of cells, development, maturation, and the sex drive. The androgens are the male sex hormones, and have masculinizing effects. Estrogens and progestogens are female sex hormones, which induce feminizing effects. Both are present at differing levels in each sex.

Interaction Between Endocrine and Nervous Systems

The endocrine and nervous systems work together to regulate the activity of many cells and tissues and maintain metabolic homeostasis in the body. The nervous system activates or inhibits target cells via electrochemical signals, in which an action potential releases neurotransmitters from the axon terminals that activate or inhibit other neurons or target cells. In contrast, endocrine cells and glands release hormones directly into the blood, which are carried throughout the body to act on specific receptors on target cells. The nervous system typically initiates very rapid responses such as reflex arcs on a time scale of milliseconds. Nervous responses both arise and fade away very quickly. The nervous and endocrine systems generally work together, but each can also operate independently. Each system can modulate or override the actions of the other.

ADRENAL GLANDS

The paired, conical adrenal glands sit atop the kidneys. Each consists of an outer cortex derived from mesoderm and an inner medulla derived from neuroectodermal neural crest cells. The chromaffin cells of the adrenal medulla are modified neurons, and are under neuronal control. The adrenal cortex secretes (1) the steroid hormones, which include the glucocorticoids, especially cortisol; and (2) the mineralocorticoids aldosterone, dehydroepiandrosterone, and androstenedione. The latter two are converted into testosterone and estrogens in the testes and the ovaries, respectively. The adrenal medulla secretes the catecholamines epinephrine and norepinephrine, which serve as both hormones and neurotransmitters. Epinephrine and norepinephrine trigger the fight-or-flight response and increase heart rate and stroke volume. They also stimulate the release of cortisol. Cortisol increases the supply of glucose and fatty acids to the brain and muscles to provide extra energy, and enhances the effects of epinephrine. Aldosterone regulates sodium and potassium levels in the blood and blood pressure via the renin-angiotensin-aldosterone system.

MAJOR ENDOCRINE GLANDS

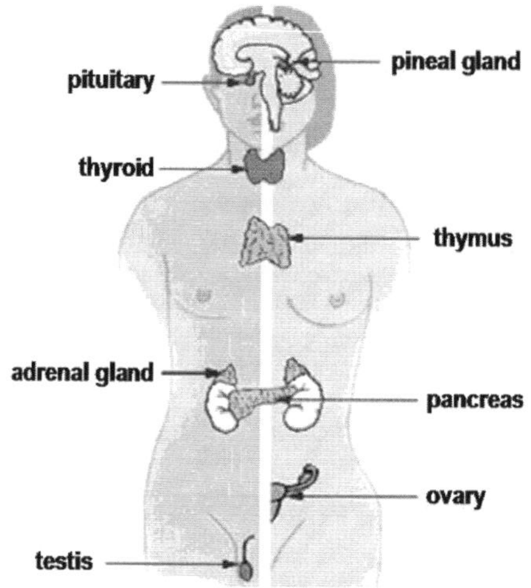

TYPES OF HORMONES

Endocrine cells and glands lack ducts, and release their chemicals directly into the bloodstream, which remain inside the body. Exocrine cells and glands are connected to ducts that carry their secretions outside the body. Sweat is excreted onto the skin, and pancreatic juice is secreted into the gut lumen (which is topologically outside the body). Hormones are released directly into the extracellular compartment or the blood. Neurohormones are released by specialized neurons into the blood rather than into a synapse like typical neurotransmitters. Classic hormones are released into the bloodstream to act on many target cells at some distance from their point of release, while autocrine hormones and paracrine hormones act locally. Paracrine hormones are released into the interstitial fluid to act on nearby target cells; autocrine hormones act on the same cells that secrete them.

Simple and Complex (Tropic) Hormonal Pathways

Simple hormone pathways are direct. An endocrine cell or a gland responds directly to a chemical or neural stimulus, and releases its hormone into the bloodstream in response to a neural or chemical stimulus. This hormone then generates a response at distant target cells, tissues, or organs. Insulin, for example, is secreted by certain cells in the pancreas in response to excess glucose in the blood. In complex, or tropic, hormone pathways, the hormone is released in response to another tropic hormone, which was secreted in response to a chemical or neural signal. Thyroid-stimulating hormone (TSH) from the adenohypophysis causes the thyroid gland to release thyroxin. In fact, TSH itself is released in response to another tropic hormone, thyroid-releasing hormone (TRH). TRH is released by the hypothalamus.

Lipid-Soluble and Water-Soluble Hormones

Water-soluble hormones activate or deactivate proteins. Their onset of action is quick, and their duration relatively short. Lipid-soluble hormones turn genes on or off. Their onset of action is slower, and their effects last much longer. In both cases, a hormone binds to its receptor, causing a signal transduction cascade that produces a cellular response. Water-soluble hormones cannot cross the plasma membrane; they bind to receptors on the cell surface, which sends a signal to the appropriate target inside the cell cytoplasm. Here, signal transduction is effected by a single messenger system involving a tyrosine kinase; or a second messenger system involving cyclic AMP, cyclic GMP, or phosphatidylinositol (PIP_2 & IP_3). Insulin is an example. Lipid-soluble hormones are carried in the plasma on a carrier protein (usually albumin). They readily cross the plasma membrane and bind to cytoplasmic or nuclear receptors inside the cell. They alter transcription and translation, and affect the expression of genes. An example is testosterone.

Aldosterone

Aldosterone is part of the renin-angiotensin-aldosterone system. When blood volume and/or pressure drops, the juxtaglomerular apparatus of the nephron secretes renin, which cleaves angiotensinogen produced by the liver into angiotensin I. Angiotensin I is then converted into angiotensin II in the lungs by angiotensin I-converting enzyme (ACE), a potent vasoconstrictor. Angiotensin II then binds to receptors in the mesangial cells in the glomeruli of the kidneys, causing the adrenal cortex to release aldosterone. Aldosterone stimulates a sodium-potassium-dependent ATPase in the distal convoluted tubules and collecting tubules in the kidneys, which promotes the resorption of Na^+ and the secretion of K^+. Aldosterone also induces the release of vasopressin from the posterior pituitary. This makes the collecting tubules permeable to water, which is then passively resorbed through osmosis into the Na^+-rich interstitial cells of the kidney. These mechanisms elevate both blood volume and pressure.

Energy Requirements of Skeletal Muscle Tissue

Resting skeletal muscle expends about 54.4 kJ/kg/day (13 kcal/kg/day), or 1.5×10^{-4} kcal/s (0.63 J/s/kg). Continuous repetitive action expends approximately 24 W plus approximately 76 W of heat. This contrasts sharply with the liver, brain, heart, and kidneys, which expend 200, 240, 400, and 400 kcal/kg/day (8.4, 10, and 16.8 MJ/kg/day), respectively. On the other hand, strenuous muscular exertion can generate 314 J/s/kg of mechanical energy. Skeletal muscle accounts for about 40 percent of total body mass in men. This percentage is slightly less for women. It also accounts for about 28 percent of total resting energy expenditure. In other words, contrary to widespread belief, most of the energy expended by the body is used to support the functioning of organs like the liver, the heart, the kidneys, and the brain, which account for only six percent of body mass.

METABOLIC CHANGES DURING EXERCISE

Exercise results in an immediate increase in O_2 consumption and CO_2 production. During aerobic metabolism, glucose and fats burn O_2 to generate ATP, which produces CO_2 and H_2O as waste products. The increased O_2 demand results in greatly enhanced cardiac output, vasodilation in the skin and working muscles, and vasoconstriction in the internal organs and non-participating muscles, which leads to a decrease in vascular resistance. Pulmonary perfusion is increased, as are minute ventilation (the total volume of gas exhaled from the lungs per minute) and alveolar ventilation. Breathing rate and tidal volume also rise. When oxygen supply can no longer meet the body's demands, anaerobic metabolism commences, in which the pyruvate resulting from glycolysis is converted into lactic acid through fermentation. This results in the production of far fewer ATP molecules, and can only be sustained for a brief period (minutes) before exhaustion and dyspnea occur.

Chemistry

Carbohydrates

Carbohydrates consist of carbon, hydrogen, and oxygen, and have the general formula $C_x(H_2O)_n$, where *x* and *n* may or may not be equal. Carbohydrates are important components of all organisms that have a wide variety of metabolic and structural functions. Simple carbohydrates are monosaccharides consisting of a single sugar molecule. Glucose, fructose, and galactose are examples. Many carbohydrates can have either a linear chain or a ring structure. Complex carbohydrates include disaccharides (two sugar molecules linked together), oligosaccharides (typically three to ten sugars), and polysaccharides (macromolecules made up of many repeated sugar units). Disaccharides include sucrose (D-glucose and D-fructose) and lactose (D-galactose and D-glucose). Monosaccharides exist in two stereoisomers. Only the right-handed (dextrorotatory) D forms occur in nature. All naturally occurring macromolecules in living organisms exist as either levorotatory (L isomers) or dextrorotatory stereoisomers, but not both.

Classifications Based on Carbon Atoms

Monosaccharides containing three carbon atoms are called trioses, those with five carbon atoms are called pentoses, ones with six carbon atoms are called hexoses, and so on. Oligosaccharides and polysaccharides consist of 3 to 10 and more than 10 repeating monosaccharide units linked by glycosidic bonds, respectively. Cellulose, starch, glycogen (so-called "animal starch"), and chitin are typical polysaccharides found in nature. They are comprised of several hundred to 10,000 or so repeating glucose units. In cellulose, the glucose units are joined by β 1,4-glycoside linkages, whose bond angles form a linear chain. Starches are joined by α 1,4-glycoside linkages, whose bond angles form a spiral chain.

Cellulose

Cellulose consists of linear glucose polymers linked by β 1,4-glycoside bonds. Cellulose is an important component of plants, and is found in the vegetables we eat. Cruciferous vegetables are particularly high in cellulose ("fiber"). Although humans cannot digest cellulose, it aids in digestive processes and promotes peristalsis and regular bowel movements.

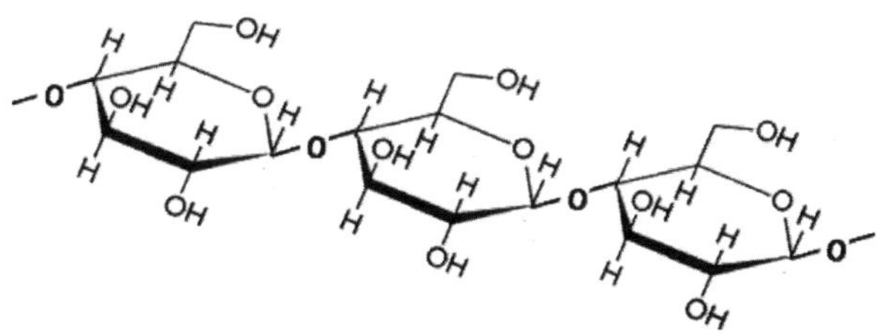

Starches

Starches are spiral glucose chains joined by α 1,4 glycoside bonds. Starch also promotes healthy digestion, and is found in many tubers, such as potatoes and carrots.

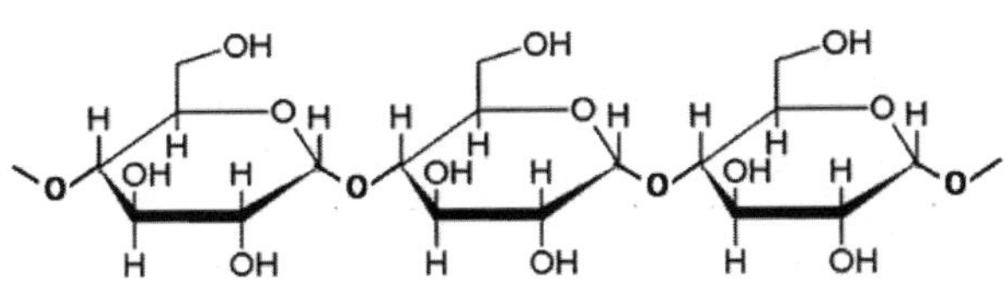

GLYCOGEN

Glycogen (so-called "animal starch") consists of multiple branching glucose units joined by α 1,4 and 1,6 glycoside linkages, and has a structure similar to starch. It is generated from glucose in the liver in response to insulin. Excess glucose is stored primarily in the liver as glycogen in response to the presence of insulin, a hormone released by the β-islet cells in the pancreas. As blood glucose levels fall during periods of fasting (such as when we sleep overnight), insulin secretion is inhibited, and the α cells of the Islets of Langerhans in the pancreas release glucagon. This stimulates glycogenolysis (the conversion of glycogen back into glucose) and gluconeogenesis to increase glucose levels in the blood.

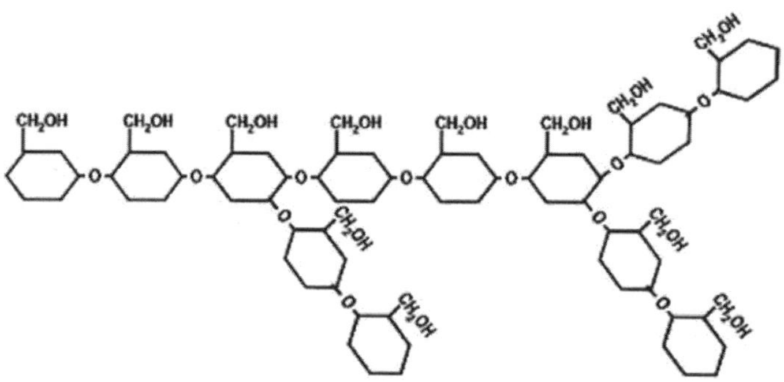

GLYCOLYSIS

Glycolysis is a cytosolic catabolic reaction in which a glucose molecule ($C_6H_{12}O_6$) is broken down into two molecules of pyruvate (pyruvic acid, CH_3COCOO^-). Two molecules of ATP (adenosine triphosphate) are generated, and two molecules of NAD^+ (nicotinamide adenine dinucleotide) are reduced to two molecules of NADH and two molecules of H^+. Two water molecules are also produced. The overall reaction is shown in the following chemical equation: $C_6H_{12}O_6$ + 2 ADP + 2 P_i + 2 NAD^+ → 2 CH_3COCOO^- + 2 ATP + 2 NADH + 2 H_2O + $2H^+$. The nine enzymatic steps of glycolysis are part of both aerobic respiration and anaerobic respiration (fermentation). Two ATP molecules are hydrolyzed into ADP in steps one and three, and four ATP molecules are generated in steps six and nine (which occur twice), yielding a net gain of two ATP molecules for every glucose molecule broken down. NAD^+ is also reduced twice to generate two NADH molecules and two protons (H^+).

Enzymatic Steps

Enzymatic steps of glycolysis:

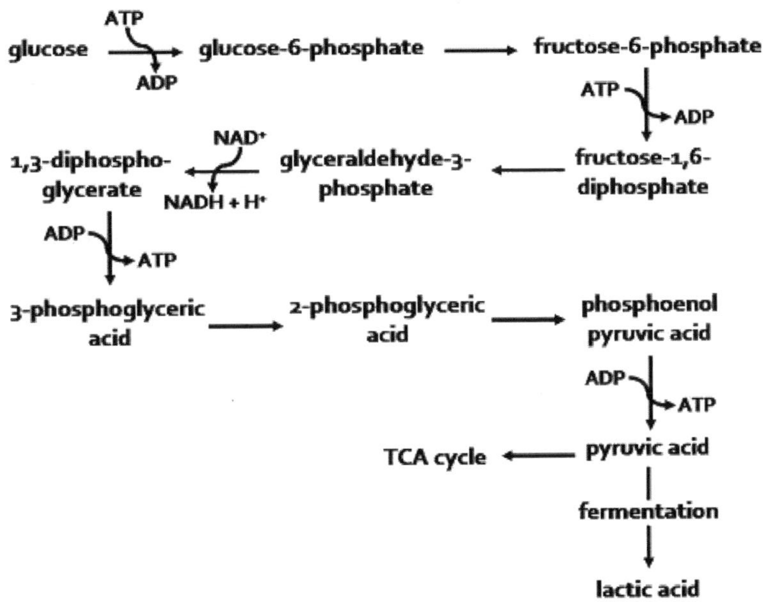

Lactic Acid Fermentation

Under anaerobic conditions, the reducing equivalents (NADH and H^+) generated in step five of glycolysis (see flashcard 7) are used to reduce two pyruvate molecules to two molecules of lactic acid in a process known as fermentation. This regenerates NAD^+, which can be shuttled back for use in step five. Lactate fermentation occurs in animal muscle when more energy is required than can be supplied by the blood. Lactate buildup after a hard workout is what makes your muscles sore. The chemical equation for this reaction is $C_6H_{12}O_6 \rightarrow 2\ CH_3COCOO^- \rightarrow 2\ CH_3CHOHCOO^-$.

Gluconeogenesis

Gluconeogenesis is the *de novo* generation of glucose in the liver during periods of fasting (such as when we sleep at night) or starvation. It is largely, but not completely, a reversal of glycolysis, in which glucose is generated from other substrates such as pyruvate, lactate, glycerol, and certain amino acids. Because step nine of glycolysis (see flashcard 7) is irreversible, pyruvate must be carboxylated into oxaloacetate inside the mitochondria in order to be converted back into PEP. This oxaloacetate must then be reduced to malate to be transported out of the mitochondria. The malate is then reoxidized to oxaloacetate in the cytoplasm, and is then decarboxylated and phosphorylated to generate PEP (phosphoenolpyruvate), which is then run backwards through the glycolytic pathway.

Aerobic Respiration

Aerobic respiration is the oxygen-requiring process that occurs in the mitochondria. During aerobic respiration, carbohydrates, fats, and proteins are broken down completely to yield energy (as ATP) and the waste products H_2O and CO_2. The preferred substrate is pyruvate derived from glycolysis in the cytosol, which must be carried across the mitochondrial membrane into the matrix, where it enters the Krebs (TCA) cycle. Here, the reducing equivalents (NADH and $FADH_2$) and protons needed to power the final stage—the chemiosmotic electron transport chain—are generated. CO_2 is also produced as a waste product. The electron transport chain is where molecular oxygen is split, ATP is generated by oxidative phosphorylation, and water is produced as a byproduct. Glycolysis and anaerobic fermentation produce a net gain of two ATP molecules from one glucose molecule. The TCA cycle and the electron transport chain can theoretically generate an additional 34 ATP molecules, but "leakage" and other factors reduce the actual gain to 29 or 30.

Lipids

Lipids are a complex group of nonpolar, hydrophobic, lipophilic molecules that include the fats, waxes, sterols, fat-soluble vitamins, acylglycerols (glycerides), and phospholipids. They are soluble in organic solvents, but insoluble or only marginally soluble in water. Since they are largely unoxidized, fats store a greater amount of metabolic energy than an equal mass of carbohydrates or proteins. Because they are nonpolar and hydrophobic, they are stored in adipocytes (animal fat storage cells) in an anhydrous state, while carbohydrates bind considerable amounts of water in similar physiological conditions. This explains why, when oxidized, fats yield much more energy than carbohydrates.

Fatty Acids

Free fatty acids (FFAs) consist of long aliphatic (non-aromatic hydrocarbon) chains with a terminal group. Their general structure is $H_3C—(CH_2)_n—COOH$. Fatty acids may be saturated (meaning they have a complete complement of hydrogen atoms) or unsaturated (meaning they have one or more C=C double bonds). A formula showing the structure of the latter is $H_3C—(CH_2)_n—HC=CH—CH_2—COOH$. Three fatty acids covalently esterified to a glycerol molecule form a triacylglycerol (triglyceride). Fats and oils (which are solid and liquid at room temperature, respectively) are triglycerides that differ in their degree of saturation. Fats tend to be saturated, while oils are unsaturated. The double carbon bonds in unsaturated fatty acids distort the linear structure seen in saturated ones. Carbon-carbon double bonds may be *cis* or *trans*. The carbon chains on either side of a *cis* bond are both oriented in either the "up" or "down" position. *Trans* bonds have carbon chains on either side of the C=C bond oriented in opposite directions.

Triglyceride Structure

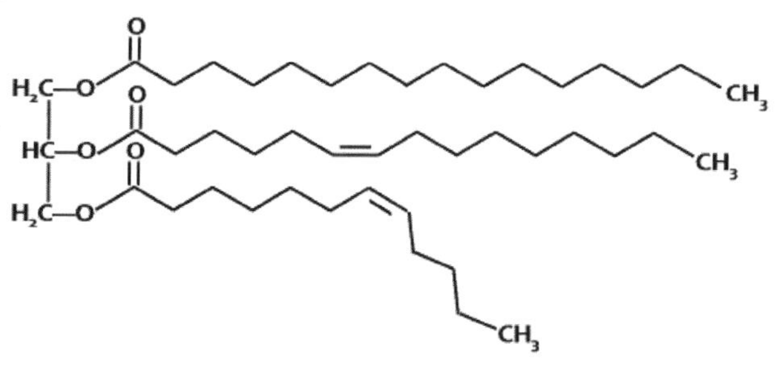

Phospholipid

Glycerophospholipids are the main components of biological membranes. They consist of a glycerol moiety esterified to two fatty acid tails and a phosphoryl (phosphate) group (see flashcard 16). Phospholipids possess two nonpolar fatty acid tails and a highly polar and water soluble phosphate head. The nature of the R group attached to the phosphate head determines the class to which a given phospholipid belongs. A phospholipid may be a phosphatidic acid, a phosphatidylglycerol, a phosphatidylcholine (lecithin), a phosphatidylinositol, or another type.

Typical phospholipid:

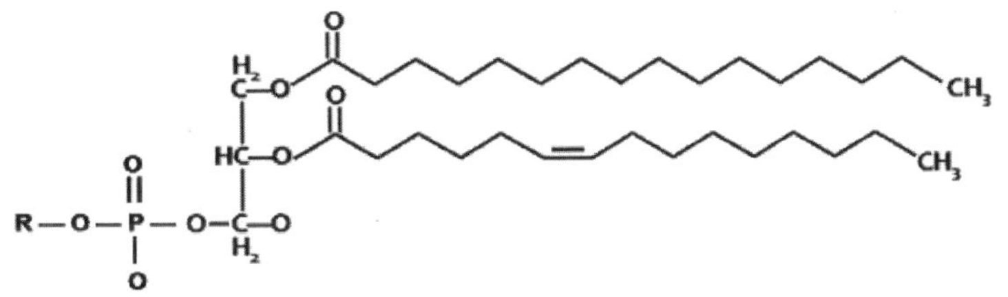

Steroids

Steroids are derived from cyclopentanoperhydrophenanthrene, a polycyclic frame consisting of four fused saturated rings. Cholesterol (shown on the right), the most abundant animal steroid, is an important component of the plasma membrane in animals. The hydroxyl (—OH) group at the C-3 position makes cholesterol weakly polar, while its fused ring system confers structural rigidity and makes it structurally important to membrane systems. Cholesterol is the basis of all steroid hormones, including cortisol and aldosterone.

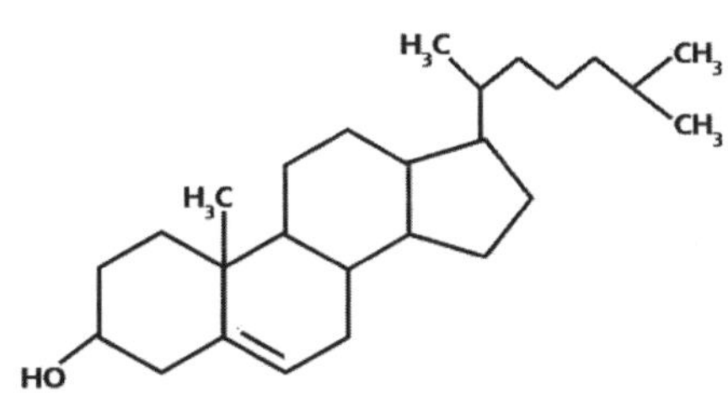

Role of Phospholipids and Cholesterol in Biological Membranes

Amphiphilic (simultaneously hydrophilic and lipophilic) molecules like phospholipids spontaneously form lipid bilayers. The hydrophobic fatty acid tails of these bilayers point inwards, while their hydrophilic phosphate heads point outwards and are in direct contact with water molecules (see flashcard 19). The orderly arrangement of these bilayers is affected by (1) the amount of unsaturation of the fatty acid tails, which distorts their packing architecture; and (2) the presence of cholesterol molecules, which pack in between the phospholipids and cause them to spread out. This tends to "fluidize" the membrane and render it less compact and rigid than it would otherwise be. This enables embedded proteins and other molecules (which further fluidize the membrane) to move about, much like a dense layer of ice cubes floating on the surface of water in a pan. This property is critical for receptors and enzymes linked to G-protein-coupled receptors.

Animal Cell Membrane

The polar phosphate heads of the phospholipids (small circles) orient toward the water molecules, while hydrophobic hydrocarbon tails point inward. Cholesterol molecules (black) inserted between the phospholipids distort the system's architecture and fluidize the bilayer. This distortion is augmented by C=C bonds, which produce kinks in the hydrocarbon chains.

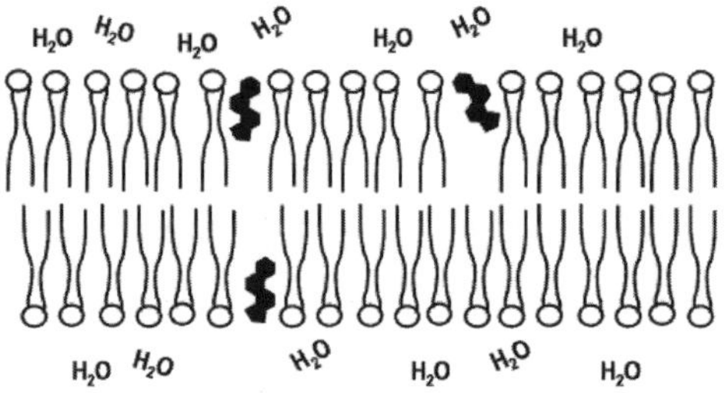

Lipogenesis

Excess dietary carbohydrates are converted to triglycerides (TGs). Free fatty acids (FFAs) are synthesized from acetyl co-A (derived from pyruvate generated by glycolysis and other processes) by fatty acid synthetase complexes. This is achieved by adding two carbon units (acyl groups) at a time. These FFAs are then esterified into TGs in the Golgi apparatus of the liver cells. They are then packaged into VLDLs for export and carried through the blood. Cholesterol synthesis begins with the formation of HMG Co-A (3-hydroxy-3-methylglutarate Co-A), which is converted into mevalonate by HMG Co-A reductase. Mevalonate then undergoes a series of condensation reactions to form lanosterol, and then cholesterol.

Catabolism of Lipids

Beta-oxidation is the four-step process by which FAs are broken down in the mitochondrial matrix to generate acetyl Co-A, which is then run through the TCA cycle. An FA in the cytosol is activated by the addition of a coenzyme-A group. This in turn reacts with carnitine to form acylcarnitine, which is carried across the mitochondrial membrane, where beta-oxidation occurs. The beta carbon of the acyl Co-A complex is then oxidized in a three-step process to produce 3-ketoacyl Co-A. The beta-ketoacyl Co-A group is then cleaved to form acetyl Co-A plus the remainder of the FA, which is combined with another coenzyme A. The process then repeats itself as needed.

Transport and Storage of Lipids

Being hydrophobic, FFAs are carried in the blood complexed to albumin. Other lipids are transported complexed to lipoproteins, which are classified according to their ratio of proteins to lipids and their densities. The FFAs arranged in order of increasing size and decreasing density (and increasing protein to lipid ratios) are chylomicrons, VLDLs, IDLs, LDLs, and HDLs. FFAs liberated from dietary fats in the intestine by lipase activity are complexed into micelles by bile salts and lecithin, and are absorbed by the epithelium of the small intestine. They are then reesterified into TGs and carried by chylomicrons to the bloodstream. There, they are again hydrolyzed to FFAs and glycerol by lipoprotein lipase. They are then absorbed by cells for energy or deposited out in adipocytes. Apolipoproteins synthesized in the liver transport cholesterol in the blood. VLDLs ("bad cholesterol") deposit their TGs in adipocytes, becoming LDLs in the process. These LDLs then carry their remaining cholesterol loads to peripheral cells, which can lead to the development of arterial plaque. HDLs ("good cholesterol") carry excess cholesterol from peripheral tissues to the liver, where it is incorporated into the bile.

Peptides and Proteins

The 20 naturally occurring amino acids are the building blocks of proteins. Some are also essential nutrients. Amino acids have the general formula $H_2NCHRCOOH$, where R is a variable side group. Amino acids have an amine group, a carboxylic acid group, and a side chain all attached to an α-

carbon atom. At physiological pH, the amino and carboxylate groups are ionized to a zwitterion, which acts as both an acid and a base.

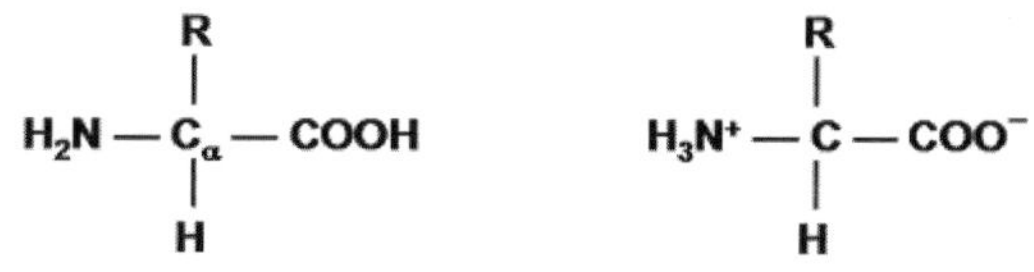

α-amino acid　　　　*Zwitterion*

PEPTIDE BONDS

Amino acids polymerize by forming a CO—NH peptide bond (see figure on the right), which is done by eliminating a water molecule. Depending on their length, these linear chains are known as peptides, polypeptides, or proteins. Peptides can have fewer than 10 amino acid residues, while polypeptides can have 40 or more. Proteins can contain more than 4,000 amino acid residues, and have molecular masses of nearly 450 kDa.

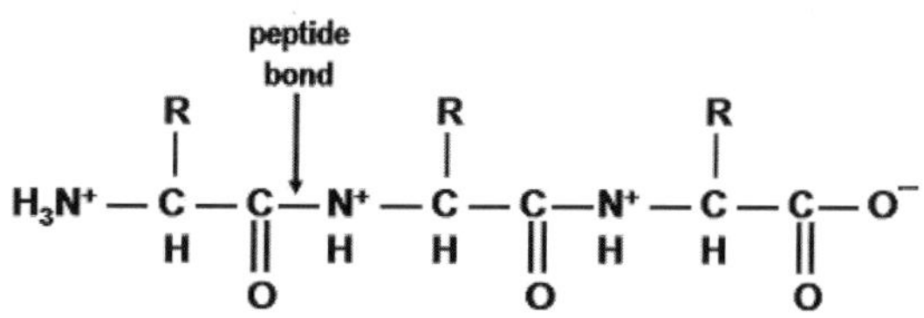

STRUCTURE OF PROTEIN

PRIMARY STRUCTURE

The primary structure of a polypeptide or protein is its amino acid sequence (i.e. its linear arrangement of amino acids). The two ends of the chain are called the carboxyl terminus (C-terminus) and the amino terminus (N-terminus).

SECONDARY STRUCTURE

The distribution of ionic charges and other noncovalent interactions such as van der Waals forces and hydrogen bonds cause polypeptides to spontaneously assume regular, secondary folded structures characterized by alpha helices and beta-pleated sheets.

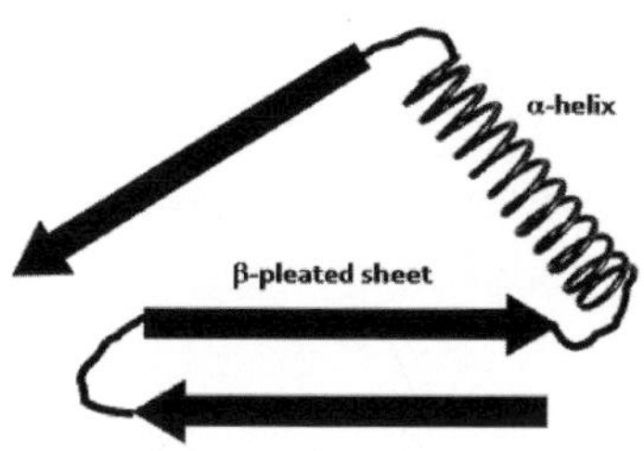

TERTIARY STRUCTURE

The tertiary structure of a protein is its overall three-dimensional configuration. This is determined by the burial of hydrophobic residues away from water, and is secured by electrostatic salt bridges and hydrogen and disulfide bonds (R—S—S—R). Examples of protein tertiary structures are shown below.

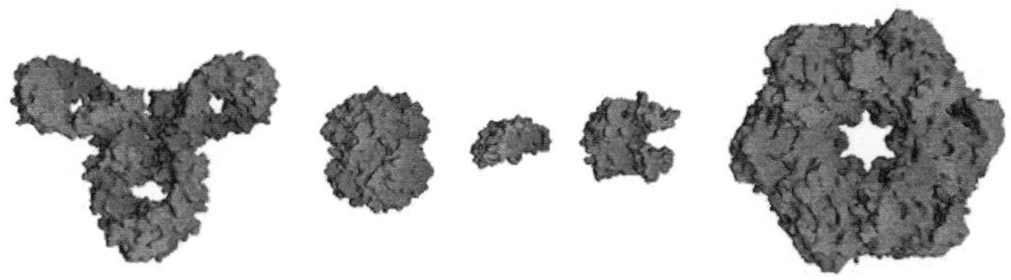

*Structures from the Protein Data Bank.

Quaternary Structure

The assembly of two or more protein subunits into multimeric complexes constitutes a protein's quaternary structure. These assemblies are stabilized by the same types of noncovalent interactions as the tertiary structure. Assemblies of two subunits constitute a dimer, three a trimer, four a tetramer, and so forth. Hemoglobin (shown on the right) is an example of a tetramer that incorporates two α and two β subunits.

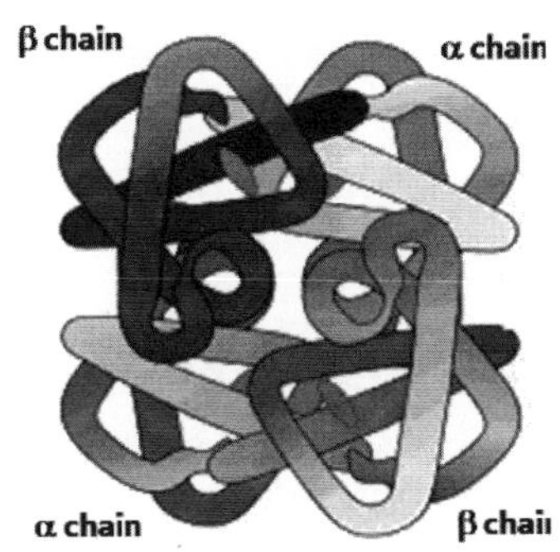

Functions of Proteins

Proteins and peptides have functions related to every aspect of cell biology and organismic physiology. They provide structural support (e.g., collagen, elastin, and keratin), allow for movement (e.g., contractile proteins like actin and myosin), play some role in nearly every biochemical process (all enzymes are proteins), and aid in immunity (antibodies). They also aid in transport (e.g., hemoglobin, lipoproteins, and cytochromes) and storage, and support hormone structure and function. Mutational changes in protein amino acid sequences are the primary vehicles underlying micro- and macroevolution.

Enzyme

An enzyme is a protein that catalyzes specific biochemical reactions or classes of reactions by lowering the activation energy of the reaction. The enzyme itself is unchanged by the process. Enzymes interact with a reactant (the substrate) to produce one or more products. Most enzymatic reactions proceed a million times or more faster than they would if they were not catalyzed. Enzyme reactions take place in two stages: (1) the enzyme (E) reversibly binds with the substrate (S) to form an enzyme-substrate complex (ES); and (2) the enzyme then catalyzes the reaction and releases the product (P), and the enzyme emerges unchanged. As shown by the double arrows in the equation below showing an enzymatic reaction, many (but not all) enzymatic reactions are reversible.

$$E + S \leftrightarrow ES \leftrightarrow E + P$$

Classification

An enzyme is named by adding the suffix "-ase" to the name of the substrate or class of substrates on which it acts. Thus, proteases, lipases, and amylases catalyze the breakdown of proteins, lipids, and starches, respectively. Sucrase catalyzes the breakdown of sucrose into fructose and glucose. Oxidase-dehydrogenases are involved in oxidation-reduction reactions, transferases transfer functional groups from one molecule to another, polymerases catalyze the formation of biological polymers, and so forth. Some enzymes were named before the current nomenclatural system was put in place. Examples include pepsin, trypsin, and chymotrypsin, which are digestive enzymes that catalyze the hydrolysis of proteins. Some proteases are secreted in an inactive form known as a proenzyme or zymogen to prevent destruction of the secreting glands. Zymogens are commonly named by attaching the suffix "-inogen" to the enzyme's root. Thus, pepsinogen is the zymogen of pepsin, chymotrypsinogen is the zymogen of chymotrypsin, and so forth.

Lock-and-Key Model of Enzyme Action

A typical enzymatic reaction is shown on the right. (1) The enzyme has a high affinity for the substrate. (2) The enzyme binds reversibly with the substrate. (3) The enzyme releases the reaction products, and is ready to bind to another substrate molecule. An enzyme often undergoes a slight conformational shift to accommodate the reaction, but it immediately resumes its original configuration once the reaction is complete. It can then bind to another substrate molecule.

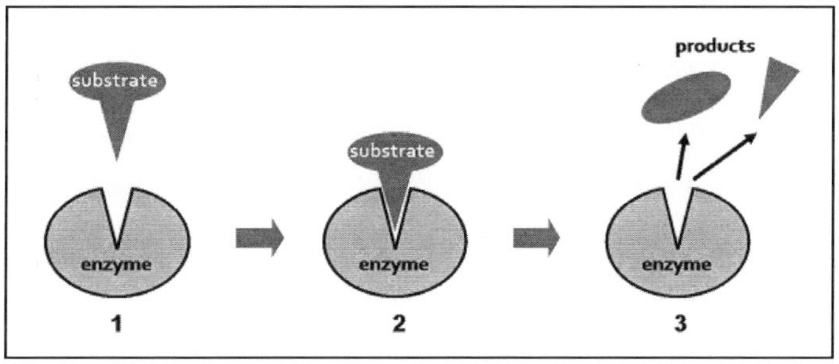

Cofactors and Coenzymes in Enzymatic Reactions

Many enzymes require nonprotein cofactors or protein coenzymes to become fully functional. Cofactors include inorganic metal ions (e.g., Ca^{2+} and Mg^{2+}) and organic compounds, such as tightly bound prosthetic groups (e.g., heme and flavin) and loosely bound coenzymes (e.g., NAD^+, $NADP^+$, FAD, and the like). Coenzymes transport functional groups (e.g., protons, hydride ions, phosphate groups, and methyl and acetyl groups) from one molecule to another. Coenzymes are often derived from vitamins (e.g., thiamine and folic acid). Coenzymes are chemically changed during enzymatic reactions, and may be regarded as a type of substrate. For example, NAD^+ and NADH are interconvertibly reduced and oxidized back and forth into each other, as is shown in the following equations: $NAD^+ \leftrightarrow NADH + H^+$, $NADP^+ \leftrightarrow NADPH + H^+$, $FAD \leftrightarrow FADH_2$, and $ATP \leftrightarrow ADP$. Apoenzyme refers to the inactive polypeptide or protein portion of an enzyme without its coenzyme; the fully functional enzyme-cofactor complex is called a holoenzyme.

Enzyme Kinetics

Enzymatic reactions exhibit saturation kinetics. For a given enzyme concentration, the rate of reaction increases rapidly with increasing substrate concentration, as this increases the rate at which the substrate and the enzyme encounter each other. This statement holds true only up to a certain point, however. The rate of reaction tapers off as substrate concentrations become very high. It asymptotically approaches the theoretical maximum for that particular enzyme concentration, V_{max}, as the enzyme active sites become saturated (see figure on the right). The Michaelis-Menten constant, K_M, is the substrate concentration necessary for the reaction to proceed at one-half its maximum rate ($\frac{1}{2}V_{max}$). K_M and V_{max} are the constants that describe enzyme kinetics.

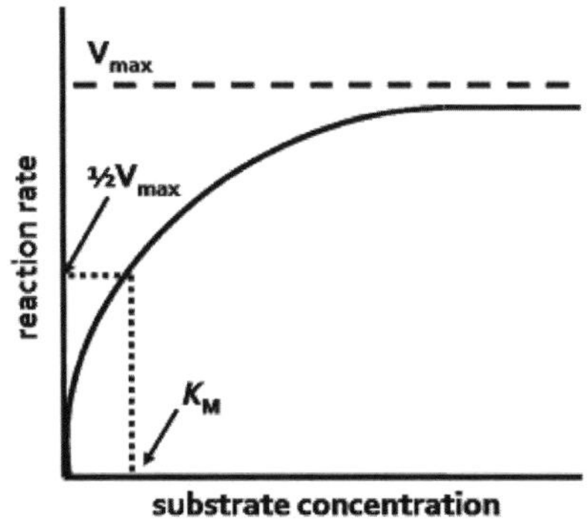

Rate Constants and Zero-Order, First-Order, and Second-Order Enzyme Kinetics

Rate constants are proportionality constants that connect reaction rates and substrate concentrations. Every reaction has specific rate constants that are directly related to the equilibrium constant for that reaction. Most enzymatic reactions are reversible. At equilibrium, the forward reaction rate equals the back reaction rate. In other words, A → B = B → A. The equilibrium constant is expressed as $k_{eq} = \frac{k_1}{k_{-1}} = \frac{[B]}{[A]}$. The brackets indicate the molar concentrations of the reactants.

A brief overview of zero-order, first-order, and second-order reactions is presented below:

- Zero-order (rate = k, reaction rate is independent of substrate concentration [S])
- First-order (rate = k[S], reaction rate is proportional to the first power of [S])
- Second-order (rate = $k[S]^2$, reaction rate is proportional to the square of the concentration of the substrate)

Enzyme Regulation and Inhibition

Enzyme inhibitors bind to enzymes and decrease or block their activity. Inhibitors can be reversible or irreversible. Irreversible inhibitors usually bind covalently to an enzyme and change it chemically in some way, commonly by altering key amino acid residues. Reversible inhibitors bind non-covalently to the enzyme, to the enzyme-substrate complex, or to both by means of hydrogen bonds, ionic bonds, and/or hydrophobic interactions. Enzymes in metabolic pathways are often inhibited by the buildup of downstream products in a negative feedback mechanism. Competitive inhibitors compete directly with the substrate for the catalytic (active) site, and inhibition can be reversed by increasing the substrate concentration or decreasing the concentration of the inhibitor. These inhibitors can bind to the enzyme, but not to the enzyme-substrate complex.

COMPETITIVE ENZYME INHIBITION

(1) The competitive inhibitor typically has a greater affinity for the catalytic site than the substrate does. (2) The inhibitor binds to the catalytic site and prevents the substrate from docking.

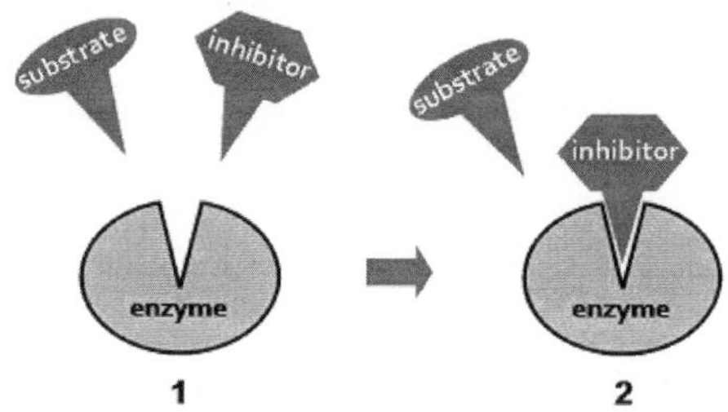

NONCOMPETITIVE INHIBITION

Noncompetitive inhibitors bind to the enzyme or enzyme-substrate complex at a site other than the catalytic site, as shown in the diagram on the right. This either blocks the substrate from binding or prevents the enzyme-substrate complex from generating the product(s). This inhibition cannot be reversed by adding substrate.

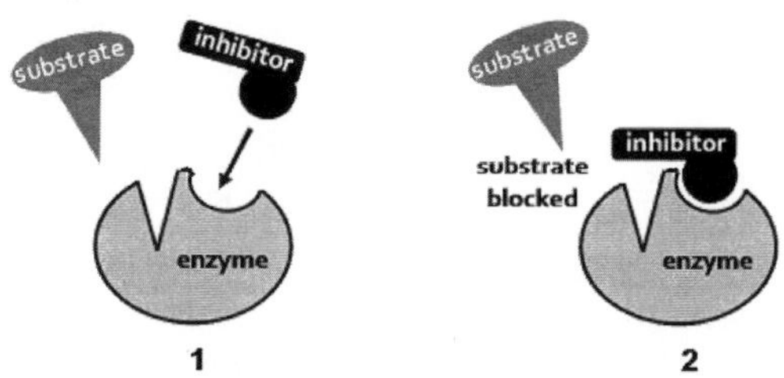

HORMONES

A hormone is a chemical substance released by a cell or a gland in one part of the body that is transported in the blood. It acts as a signal at one or more specific, distant target receptors, cells, or organs. Endocrine hormones are released directly into the bloodstream, whereas exocrine hormones are secreted into a duct. From here, they enter the blood or diffuse out to act upon neighboring cells or tissues. Endocrine hormones in particular cooperate with the central, peripheral, and enteric nervous systems to regulate homeostasis, cell division, and development. Hormones can be peptides or glycoproteins derived from lipids or phospholipids, or from monoamines. They may also function as neurotransmitters in the nervous system.

MAJOR CLASSES OF HORMONES

Hormones fall into three major classes: amine hormones, peptide and protein hormones, and steroid hormones. Amine hormones are derived from one of two amino acids: tyrosine (epinephrine and norepinephrine) or tryptophan (melatonin and serotonin). These hormones also serve as neurotransmitters. Amine hormones are water soluble, and are readily carried in the blood. They activate membrane-bound G protein-coupled receptors. Melatonin, however, is also lipid soluble, and binds to nuclear receptors inside the cell as well. Peptide- and protein-derived hormones are likewise water soluble, and travel freely in the blood. The third class of hormones is built upon a steroid frame. Lipid-soluble steroid hormones are derived from cholesterol, and require a carrier protein—primarily albumin—for transport in the blood. Water-soluble hormones simply switch protein receptors on or off. They have a quick onset, and their duration of action is short. Lipid-soluble hormones switch genes on or off. Their onset is slower than that of water-soluble hormones, and their duration of action is longer.

Classic, Autocrine, and Paracrine Hormones and Neurohormones

Classic hormones are released directly into the bloodstream. They travel throughout the body to act on many target cells, often at some distance from their point of release. Paracrine hormones are released into the interstitial fluid to act on nearby target cells. Autocrine hormones act on the same cells that secrete them. Neurohormones are released directly into the blood by specialized neurons called neurosecretory or neuroendocrine cells. Most neurons release neurotransmitter chemicals into a synapse.

Direct and Tropic Hormonal Control Pathways

The pathways from the release of a hormone to its effect at a distant target cell or tissue may be simple or complex. Simple hormone pathways are direct. An endocrine cell or gland responds directly to a chemical or neural stimulus by releasing its hormone into the bloodstream. The hormone then travels to its distant target cells, tissues, or organs to produce the desired response. For example, insulin is secreted by certain cells in the pancreas in response to excess plasma glucose. In a complex or tropic hormone pathway, the hormone is released in response to another hormone called a tropic hormone. A tropic hormone is secreted in response to a chemical or neural signal. Thyroid-stimulating hormone (TSH), which causes the thyroid to release thyroxin, is an example. TSH is itself released in response to yet another tropic hormone, thyrotropin-releasing hormone (TRH), which is secreted by the pituitary.

Nucleotide

The nitrogenous nucleobase (in this case adenine) is attached to a pentose (in this case ribose, which is encircled by the dotted line) at the C-1 position, forming a nucleoside. The phosphate is attached to the sugar at C-5; the entire complex constitutes a nucleotide. The addition of two additional phosphate groups would form adenosine triphosphate (ATP), the main energy-carrying molecule in animals.

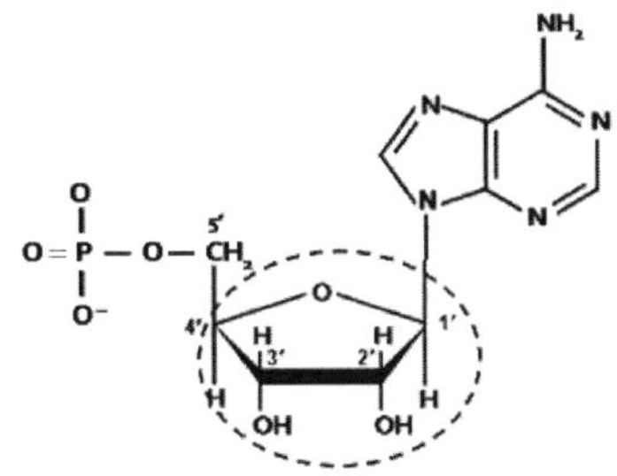

Nucleic Acids

Nucleotides join together to form the nucleic acids DNA and RNA. They also play a major role in various metabolic processes. Adenosine triphosphate (ATP) and guanosine triphosphate (GTP) carry chemical energy in their attached phosphate groups, and as cyclic monophosphates (cAMP and cGMP) are important in cellular signal transduction. Single nucleotides are also components of critical enzymatic cofactors such as nicotinamide adenine dinucleotide (NAD^+) and flavin adenine dinucleotide (FAD), which function in redox reactions. They are important components of coenzyme A (co-A), which is a critical cofactor in the synthesis and β oxidation of fatty acids and in the oxidation of pyruvic acid in the tricarboxylic acid (TCA) cycle.

Metabolism of Nucleic Acids

Dietary and tissue nucleic acids are catabolized by pancreatic and lysosomal enzymes, respectively. The protein moiety is then broken down into its constituent amino acids and metabolized normally. Nucleic acids are split into mononucleotides by phosphodiesterases, which are hydrolyzed to their constituent nucleosides and inorganic phosphate by nucleotidases. Purines are converted in the liver into uric acid, which is then excreted by the kidneys. Pyrimidines are converted into beta amino acids, ammonia, and CO_2.

ATP

ATP (adenosine triphosphate) is formed by adding two phosphate groups to adenine. An ATP molecule contains three phosphate groups, and is produced from adenosine diphosphate (ADP) or adenosine monophosphate (AMP) by ATP synthase. ATP powers energy-requiring reactions by giving up a phosphate group and converting back into one of its precursors. ATP releases energy when the pyrophosphate linkage between two phosphate groups is hydrolyzed, either by removing the terminal phosphate to form ADP or by removing the terminal diphosphate to form AMP and pyrophosphate.

DNA and RNA

Nucleic acid is the general term for ribonucleic acid (RNA) and deoxyribonucleic acid (DNA). Nucleic acids code for and function in the transcription and translation of genetic information into proteins. Nucleotides consist of a pentose, or five-carbon sugar (either ribose or 2′-deoxyribose), a nitrogen-containing nucleobase, and a phosphate group. They are the building blocks of nucleic acids. A nucleobase and a pentose together comprise a nucleoside; the addition of a phosphate forms a nucleotide. Ribose (see flashcard 44) has a hydroxyl group (—OH) at C-2; deoxyribose has a hydrogen atom at that position.

RNA (ribonucleic acid) and DNA (deoxyribonucleic acid) consist of very long nucleotide polymers whose alternating pentose and phosphate groups (the backbone of the nucleic acid) are linked by phosphodiester bonds (see flashcard 48). RNA has two hydrogen atoms at the 2-carbon position; DNA has a hydrogen and a hydroxyl group. Eukaryotic DNA consists of two antiparallel strands whose nucleobases are hydrogen bonded to their complementary counterparts on the opposite strand. Each antiparallel strand terminates in a phosphate group at the 5′ end and in a hydroxyl group at the 3′ end. Two types of nucleobases exist: pyrimidines and purines. The four nucleobases in DNA are the purines adenine (A) and guanine (G), and the pyrimidines thymine (T) and cytosine (C). Uracil (U) is substituted for thymine in RNA. In opposite strands of nucleic acids, purines form base pairs with pyrimidines. A always pairs with T, while G pairs with C. Base pairs are cross linked by hydrogen bonds.

Base Pairing Relationships

Base pairing relationships between C and G and T and A

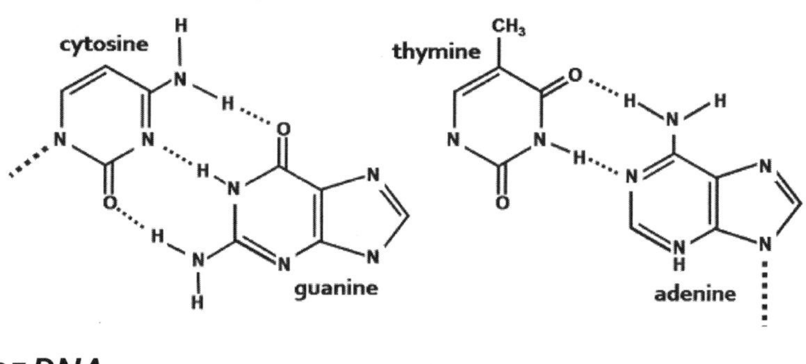

Basic Structure of DNA

DNA exists *in vivo* as a double helix with two complementary strands wound around each other in an α-helical spiral. Because of complementary base pairing relationships, cytosine and adenine form three hydrogen bonds with each other, while adenine and thymine form only two. DNA is also directional. A 5′ to 3′-oriented strand pairs with one running in the opposite direction: 3′ to 5′. Nucleic acid replication occurs from 5′ to 3′, whereas transcription runs from 3′ to 5′. Complexed with histones, DNA normally exists as a long, tightly coiled sequence packaged in a chromosome containing millions of base pairs and thousands of individual genes. Each end of a chromosome (or of the sister chromatids) is capped by a protective sequence of repetitive DNA known as a telomere.

Basic Structure of a Gene

Genes have one or more promoters—regulatory sequences that facilitate transcription—that are usually located "upstream" (i.e. at the 5′ end) of the remainder of the gene. Various enhancer sequences may also be present to help initiate transcription. As shown below, these regulatory sequences are followed by a series of exons (expressed regions, or coding sequences) and introns (intragenic regions, which are deleted in the mature mRNA transcript), up to the terminator sequence.

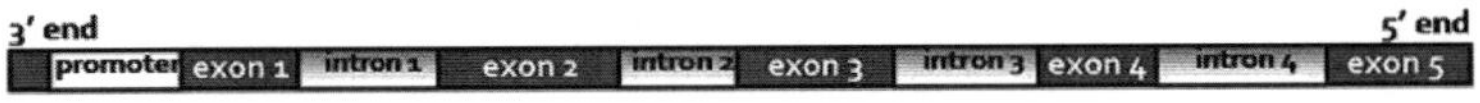

Transcription

DNA transcription involves three main steps: (1) RNA polymerase binds to specific DNA nucleotide sequences in the promoter area of the gene to be transcribed. Other sequences tell the enzyme where to begin and end transcription. (2) Transcription factors unwind the DNA strand and allow the RNA polymerase to attach the antisense strand, which is the one serving as the template to be transcribed. The untranscribed strand is the sense strand. A single DNA sequence (gene) can be simultaneously transcribed by many RNA polymerases. (3) RNA polymerase moves along the DNA antisense sequence toward the 5′ end, transcribing it into its complementary RNA chain until the terminator sequence, where it detaches from the DNA as newly transcribed mRNA. This primary mRNA transcript is then posttranscriptionally modified to excise all the introns and splice the remaining exons together. A methylated guanine cap is also added to the 5' end, and a poly-A tail is added to the 3′ end to form mature mRNA.

Translation

In eukaryotes, the newly transcribed mRNA leaves the nucleus through one of the nuclear pores and enters the cytoplasm, where the ribosomal subunits are assembled to form a functional ribosomal complex. This typically takes place on the outer membrane of the rough endoplasmic reticulum, where the mRNA/ribosomal complex usually binds. The ribosomal complex induces the complementary anticodons of transfer RNAs (each of which are attached to a specific amino acid by the 3′ CCA-terminal group) to bind to the corresponding 3-nucleobase codon on the mRNA. Thus, the codon ACC on a tRNA carrying tryptophan (Trp) would temporarily bind to the anticodon UGG on the mRNA (remember that uracil replaces thymine in RNA). The amino acids are joined together by peptide bonds in a growing peptide chain as the mRNA passes through and the ribosome "reads" each anticodon in sequence.

Basic Structure of tRNA

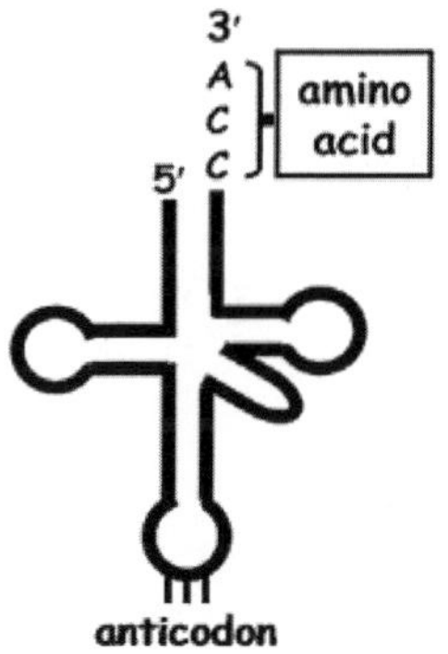

Genetic Mutations

A mutation is any error in DNA replication resulting in a mistaken substitution, insertion, or deletion of a nucleobase in a gene. Mutations also occur during meiosis when nondisjunction events prevent the normal migration of sister chromosomes to opposite poles of the cell. This can result in genetic defects such as trisomy 21 (Down's syndrome), in which the individual has three copies of chromosome 21. Translocations of segments between nonhomologous chromosomes and chromosome breakage also constitute mutations. Mutations can be caused by a variety of environmental factors: ionizing radiation, chemicals, viruses, and transposons. The latter term refers to sequences of DNA that move from one position to another within a genome by means of "copy and paste" or "cut and paste."

Vitamins

A vitamin is any water- or lipid-soluble organic compound that cannot be synthesized in adequate amounts by the body. Certain vitamins must be supplemented in the diet under certain circumstances. Examples include biotin in cases of metabolically induced deficiencies of biotin-dependent carboxylases, and vitamin D in the absence of adequate sunlight exposure. Dietary inorganic minerals and essential fatty acids and amino acids are not included in the definition of vitamins. Vitamins can function as hormones, antioxidants, precursors, or enzyme cofactors.

13 Essential Vitamins

The 13 essential vitamins are retinol (vitamin A), thiamine (B_1), ascorbate (C), calciferol (D), riboflavin (B_2), tocopherol (E), cobalamin (B_{12}), phylloquinone (K_1), pantothenic acid (B_5), biotin (B_7), pyridoxine (B_6), niacin (B_3), and folic acid (B_9). Vitamin K_2 (menaquinone) is synthesized by the gut microflora, but in some cases may need to be augmented through dietary sources. The vitamins listed above can be obtained from (among other foods) cod liver oil (A and D); rice bran (B_1); fresh foods and fruits (C); meat, dairy products, and eggs (B_2, B_3, B_5, B_6, B_7); wheat germ oil and unrefined vegetable oils (E); liver and other animal products (B_{12}); and leafy vegetables (B_9, K_1). Excess levels of certain vitamins can be toxic.

Oxidation-Reduction (Redox) Reactions

Oxidation and reduction always occur together in a redox reaction. Oxidation involves the loss of one or more electrons by an atom, an ion, or a molecule; reduction is the gain of one or more electrons by an atom, an ion, or a molecule. Redox reactions involve a redox pair: a reductant (reducing agent) and an oxidant (oxidizing agent). The reductant loses electrons, and is thereby oxidized; the oxidant gains electrons, and is thereby reduced.

Energy-Carrying Molecules in the Body

Adenosine triphosphate (ATP) and guanosine triphosphate (GTP) are pyrimidine and purine nucleoside triphosphates that carry chemical energy in their attached phosphate groups. ATP and GTP are generated by phosphorylation during cellular respiration, and both are converted back into their diphosphate precursors (ADP and GDP) when used in energy-requiring and signal transduction reactions. ATP and GTP are continually recycled between ADP and GDP by biochemical reactions in the body.

Krebs Cycle

The Krebs cycle is the first stage in oxidative cellular respiration. Two pyruvate molecules resulting from glycolysis or other catabolic processes in the cytoplasm are transported across the mitochondrial membrane. Each loses a CO_2 and becomes a two-carbon acetyl group, which combines with coenzyme-A to form acetyl co-A. Each acetyl co-A group enters the TCA (Krebs) cycle in the matrix of the mitochondria. Here, a four-carbon acid (oxaloacetate) is combined with the acetyl group to produce a six-carbon acid (citrate). This substrate then successively loses CO_2 to become first a five-carbon acid (ketoglutarate), and then a four-carbon acid again (succinate). Succinate is first oxidized to fumarate and then to oxaloacetate, and the entire process is repeated. The end result of the TCA cycle is the production of reducing equivalents ($NADH + H^+$ and $FADH_2$), which will drive the next stage: the electron transport chain.

Electron Transport Chain in Animals

The electron transport chain occurs on the inner mitochondrial membrane. In this process driven by NADH and H^+ generated in the Krebs cycle, protons are pumped into the intermembrane space, and their associated electrons are kicked up into high energy states by various electron acceptor proteins. These electrons are then allowed to cascade downhill, energetically speaking, from one electron acceptor to another. This occurs until an oxygen molecule is split to produce a water molecule. Water and carbon dioxide are the waste products of oxidative respiration. The energy of the boosted electrons pumps additional protons into the intermembrane space. These protons then flow down their concentration gradient through a channel in the terminal enzyme, ATP synthase, and the energy is used to generate ATP by chemiosmosis. The net theoretical gain of ATP from one molecule of glucose via glycolysis and oxidative phosphorylation is 36 or 38 molecules of ATP. However, the actual yield is 29 or 30. The actual yield is lower because of membrane leakage and energetic loss.

Pathology

PATHOLOGY

Pathology is the study of the diagnosis and etiology, pathogenesis, morphological changes, and clinical manifestations of cells, tissues, and organs in disease states. Medical pathology is divided into two main branches. (1) Anatomical pathology is the diagnosis of disease as manifested in the gross and/or microscopic structural, immunological, and/or molecular changes in cells, tissues, organs, or the entire organism. It includes autopsies on corpses to determine the precise cause(s) of death. (2) Clinical pathology is the diagnosis of disease states through laboratory analyses of the chemical, microbiological, hematological, and molecular parameters and manifestations in body fluids, excreta, and tissues. Forensic pathology is the determination of the immediate and/or contributory cause(s) of death in cases involving criminal or civil law. It may also involve ascertaining the identity of a corpse. The related discipline of anthropological pathology involves the application of the principles of physical anthropology, human osteology, forensic entomology, and taphonomy to determine the time of and environmental circumstances surrounding an individual's death and the subsequent decay of the body.

PREPARATION OF TISSUE SAMPLES FOR MICROSCOPIC EXAMINATION

Tissues are typically fixed in 4 percent formaldehyde in phosphate buffered saline for light microscopy, and in 2.5 percent glutaraldehyde in phosphate buffered saline for electron microscopy. Intrasurgical biopsies are generally frozen, and may be subjected to antibody-linked immunofluorescent staining to ensure that a tumor margin has been excised. Tissues are subsequently dehydrated in a graded ethanol series, cleared with xylene and embedded in paraffin, sectioned with a microtome, and stained. Stains commonly employed include hematoxylin and eosin (H and E, which stains nuclei blue and cytoplasmic structures pink), safranin, O Red O, toluidine blue, silver stain, Wright's stain, and periodic acid-Schiff stain (PAS), among others. Each stain has specific staining properties for various tissue types. Perls Prussian blue stains iron deposits blue or purple, and is used to diagnose such diseases as hemochromatosis.

BLOOD AND URINE ANALYSES

Basic metabolic tests include Ca^{2+}, Na^+, K^+, Cl^-, blood urea nitrogen (BUN), CO_2, total creatinine, urinalysis, fasting glucose, and fasting lipids. Comprehensive metabolic tests add liver function tests (ALT and AST), bilirubin, and HbA1c, in addition to others. A complete blood count is often done, which includes looking at RBC, WBC, hematocrit, MCV, MCH, and other parameters. Prothrombin clotting time may be assessed under special circumstances. Endocrine panels might include TSH, total and free T4, free T3, 24-hour urine aldosterone excretion rate and/or a spot aldosterone test followed by a furosemide challenge, PAC/PRA ratio (plasma aldosterone concentration/plasma renin activity), 8:00 a.m. cortisol (or even better, a 24-hour cortisol saliva series), and catecholamine levels.

INFLAMMATION

Inflammation is a stereotypic and generalized response by the body's innate immune system to harmful stimuli, which range from ischemia, physical injury, and toxic substances, to invasion by infectious pathogens. It is what allows injurious insults to be removed and wounds to heal. Acute inflammation is brought about by the mobilization of plasma and leukocytes to the site of the injury, which elicits a cascade of inflammatory cytokines and other signals that sequester and eliminate the damaging stimuli. Chronic inflammation is a prolonged condition involving multiple rounds of simultaneous tissue destruction and healing. It produces a change in the tissue that can lead to disease states. Both acute and chronic inflammation can also result from abnormal hypersensitivity responses, such as allergies and autoimmune disorders.

Asbestosis and the Formation of Ferruginous Bodies

Asbestosis is a chronic inflammatory fibrosis of the lung parenchyma resulting from occupational asbestos inhalation. Characteristic histopathologic manifestations include ferruginous bodies and prominent interstitial fibrosis, as shown in the micrograph image. Ferruginous bodies (the structures inside the dotted circles on the micrograph) are brown inclusions in the alveolar septa that are indicative of chronic asbestos inhalation. They are derived from ferritin and hemosiderin precipitated by macrophages that ingested and attempted to digest the fibers. The presence of ferruginous bodies is associated with an elevated risk of lung cancer and malignant mesothelioma. The latter is a rare asbestos-associated cancer that develops in the lining of the internal organs, but especially in the pleura. It can also arise in the peritoneum.

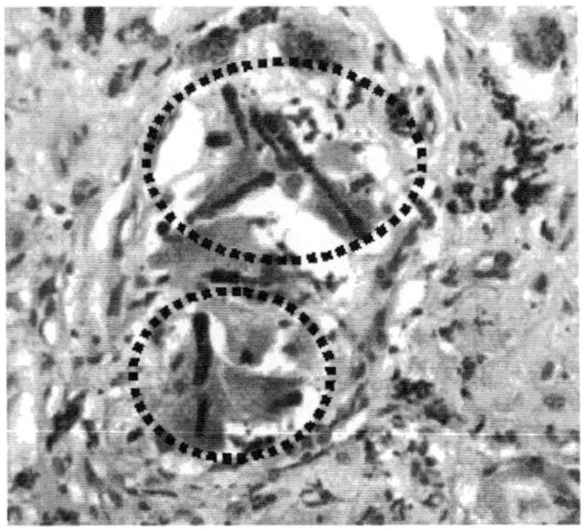

Fluid Distribution in the Body

Normally, water accounts for 60 percent of lean body mass. Of this, two-thirds is intracellular, one-third is extracellular (primarily interstitial), and about five percent is contained in the blood plasma. Edema is an abnormal accumulation of fluid in the interstitial spaces that is due to local changes in vascular permeability. Edema can result from increased hydrostatic pressure due to impaired venous outflow (e.g., in DVT) or congestive heart failure, lowered osmotic pressure resulting from excessive loss or reduced synthesis of albumin, lymphatic obstruction, sodium retention, and/or inflammation.

Volume of Distribution of a Drug

The volume of distribution of a drug (V_D) is a primary pharmacokinetic (PK) parameter. It is a factor of proportionality relating the total amount of a drug in the body (i.e. the oral or parenteral dose administered) to its measured concentration in a specific biological fluid (e.g., the plasma). V_D is equal to the total amount of a drug in the body divided by its plasma concentration. Drugs with a V_D that is equal to or less than seven liters are largely confined to the plasma. Drugs with a V_D of between 7 and 15 liters are distributed throughout the blood (plasma and formed elements). Drugs with a V_D that is greater than 42 liters are distributed through all of the body tissues, but are found in especially high levels in the fat deposits. In this last case, most of the drug is bound up in the tissues, and very little circulates in the plasma.

Clotting Cascade

Two pathways lead to fibrin formation, clot formation, and blood coagulation, which prevent exsanguination and loss of blood into or from the body. Earlier concepts explaining this process stated that the contact activation (intrinsic) pathway and the tissue factor (extrinsic) pathway, which fed into the common pathway, were equally involved in clot formation and the maintenance of hemostasis. However, it is now clear that the extrinsic pathway has a more significant role. The intrinsic pathway is activated when the blood is exposed to negatively charged surfaces; the extrinsic pathway is initiated by vascular injury, which exposes subendothelial tissue factor (factor III). In these reactions, a series comprised mainly of serine protease zymogens (FVIII and FV are glycoproteins, and factor XIII is a transglutaminase) and their glycoprotein cofactors are activated to form active enzymes that catalyze each step in the cascade. Both pathways activate the common pathway, which is comprised of factor X, thrombin, and fibrin.

Intrinsic, Extrinsic, and Common Pathways of the Clotting Cascade

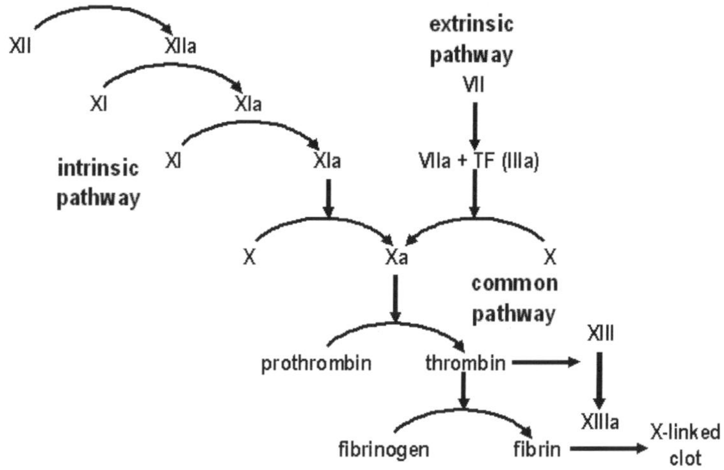

Histopathology of a Pheochromocytoma

Pheochromocytoma is a benign neuroendocrine tumor originating in the adrenal medulla that can cause sympathetic hyperactivity. Signs and symptoms include elevated pulses of catecholamines, which can produce paroxysmal (episodic) and refractory hypertension that does not respond to medication, headaches that have a sudden onset, weight loss, orthostatic hypotension, and other symptoms. The high magnification micrograph image shows a pheochromocytoma that exhibits the classic nested configuration of the cells (Zellballen) and the stippled chromatin (this accounts for the "salt-and-pepper" appearance of the chromatin inside the nuclei).

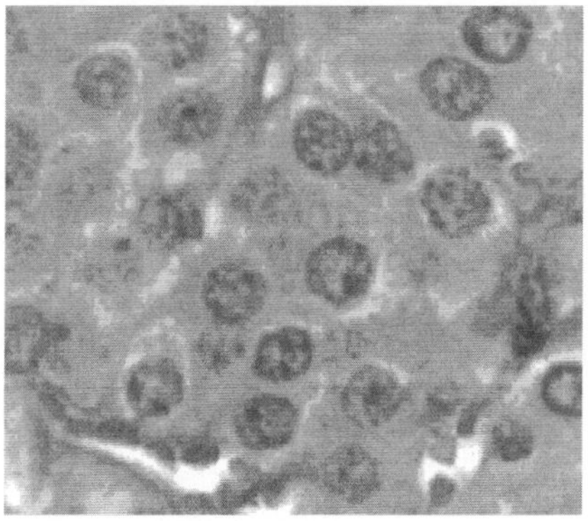

Mohs Microsurgery for Skin Cancers

Mohs surgery is the precise, microscopically controlled, surgical removal of cancerous skin tissue. It is used to achieve complete margin control while preserving as much unaffected tissue as possible. The main portion of the cancer is excised, and the margins are carefully marked. Thin layers of the margin are carefully excised in stages, and are sent to a pathologist until no cancerous cells are found. Mohs surgery has a reported five-year cure rate of 99.7 to 99.8 percent for basal cell carcinomas (94 percent for recurrent basal cell carcinomas); 94.8 percent for squamous cell cancers of the face, neck, and scalp; and 95 to 98 percent for *in situ* melanomas. Much depends on the skill and experience of the surgeon. Lower cure rates have been reported when different procedures are used.

Normal Renal Tubular Tissue and Clear Renal Cell Carcinoma

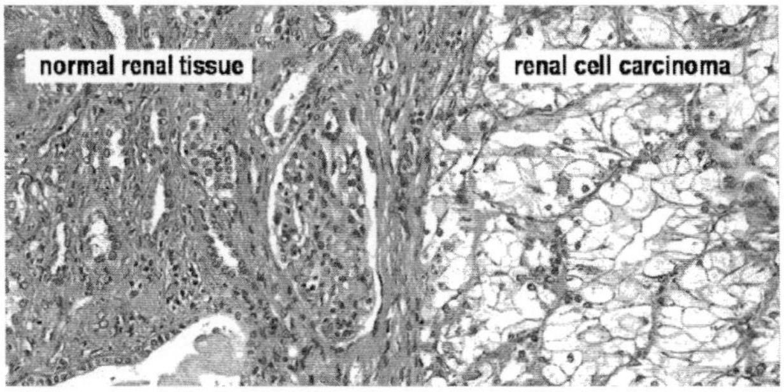

Precursor B-Cell Acute Lymphoblastic Anemia and Normal Human Blood Smear

Contrasts the appearance of precursor B-cell acute lymphoblastic anemia with that of a normal human blood smear:

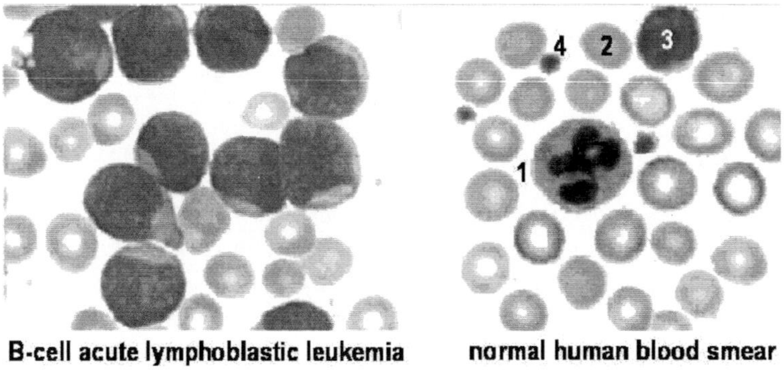

1, neutrophil; 2, red blood cell; 3, monocyte; 4, platelet

ACUTE GLOMERULAR THROMBOTIC MICROANGIOPATHY

Acute glomerular thrombotic microangiopathy in the kidney as seen in disseminated intravascular coagulopathy (DIC):

*The dotted rectangle outlines a thrombus in the hilus of a renal glomerulus.

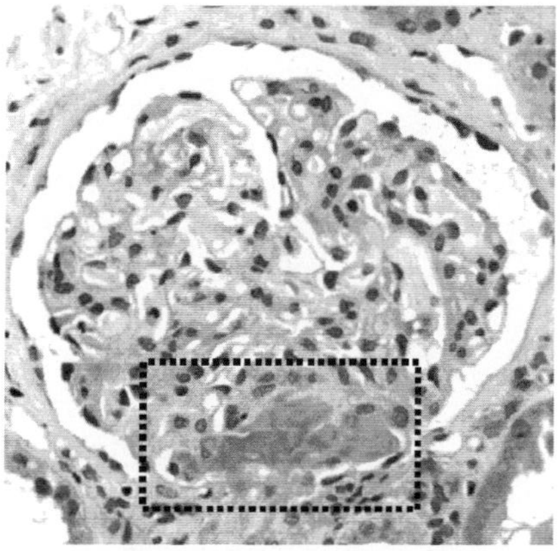

HISTOPATHOLOGICAL CHANGES IN A MYOCARDIAL INFARCTION

Contraction band necrosis (extra thick, intensely eosin staining striae) is an uncontrolled type of necrosis seen in cardiac tissue following an MI. It is due to rupture of the sarcolemma resulting from subsequent reperfusion following hypercontraction during an infarct. Karyolysis (loss of nuclei) results from the breakdown of chromatin and enucleation of the myocytes, which stain evenly with eosin. Here, the myocytes are also extensively pervaded by white fibrous scar tissue, which forms in the days following an MI as dead muscle tissue is removed by neutrophils and macrophages. This characteristic damage to myocytes is the result of ischemic damage followed by subsequent reperfusion and repair.

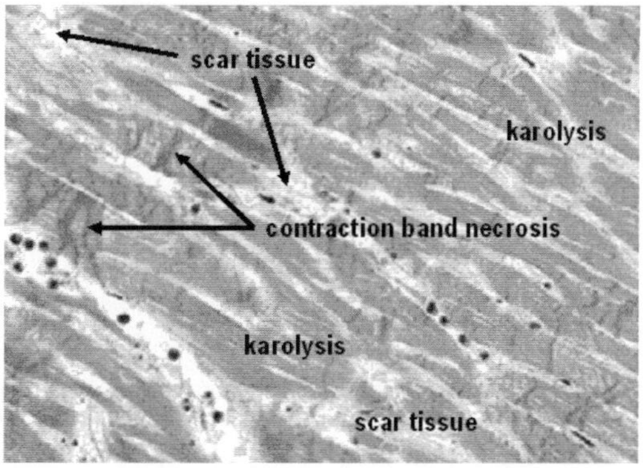

ENTAMOEBA HISTOLYTICA INFECTION

Identification of the cysts or trophozoites of *Entamoeba histolytica* in fecal specimens through the use of light microscopy used to be the classical diagnostic method for *Entamoeba histolytica* infection. However, *E. dispar*, a nonpathogenic and much more common species, is morphologically indistinguishable from *E. histolytica*. This resulted in a vast overestimate of the incidence of *E. histolytica* infections in humans—nearly 10 percent of the world's population. Then, it was discovered that 90 percent of these amoebic infections are actually due to *E. dispar*. Preliminary diagnoses based on microscopic examination of stool samples are now confirmed by radioimmunoassay (RIA) and enzyme-linked immunosorbent assay (ELISA), which detect specific *E. histolytica* antigens. Reverse line blot hybridization assay is an additional diagnostic tool that was recently introduced. The micrograph on the right (courtesy of the CDC) shows a cyst of *E. histolytica* stained with chlorazol black. The trophozoites live only a few hours outside of the host, and are destroyed by the low pH of the stomach if they are ingested. Only the cysts are infectious.

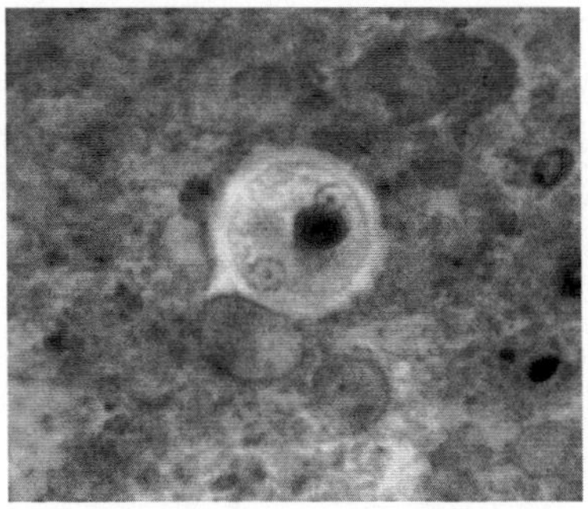

Blood Smear for Malaria

Immediate (within hours) microscopic examination of a patient's blood smear is the gold standard diagnostic procedure when dealing with suspected malaria. The smear is usually stained with Giemsa, which permits visual determination of the different species of malarial parasites. Wright's stain can be substituted as necessary when Giemsa is not available, but species determination is more problematic. Both thick and thin blood smears should be used. Thick smears permit examination of a greater volume of blood, and make detection of low-level infection that might be missed in a thin smear more likely. However, a thin smear better reveals the features of the parasite, and permits accurate differential diagnosis so the species can be determined. Four species of *Plasmodium* cause malaria in humans: *P. falciparum*, *P. vivax*, *P. ovale*, and *P. malariae*. *Plasmodium falciparum* causes the most dangerous and lethal type of malaria, and is the predominant form in Sub-Saharan Africa. The micrograph image shows ring forms and gametocytes of *Plasmodium falciparum* in human blood.

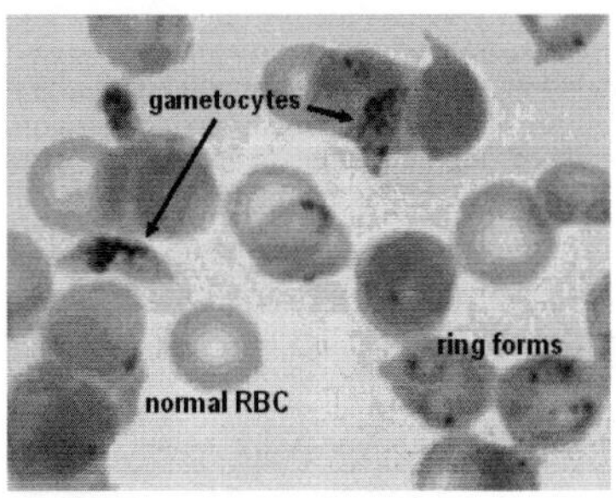

Blood Smear for Trypanosomiasis Infections

Two species of *Trypanosoma* (a kinetoplastid protozoan parasite) cause serious and often fatal diseases in humans. They can be distinguished in a blood smear through the use of light microscopy. *Trypanosoma brucei* causes African trypanosomiasis (sleeping sickness), which is widespread throughout Sub-Saharan Africa. Infections are transmitted through the bites of the tsetse fly (*Glossina* spp.). American trypanosomiasis (Chagas disease) is caused by *Trypanosoma cruzi*, which is transmitted through the bites of "assassin bugs" (Hemiptera: Reduviidae). It is widespread throughout Mexico, Central America, and South America. As with malaria, a diagnosis is made through microscopic examination of blood smears. *Trypanosoma brucei* parasites are shown in the micrograph image of a human blood smear.

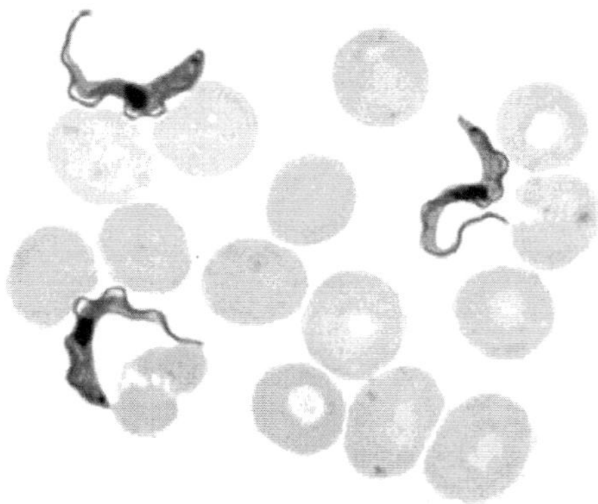

Liver Cirrhosis

Liver cirrhosis is the destruction of liver tissue due to chronic inflammation and necrosis. This tissue is replaced by fibrotic scar tissue and regenerative lumpy nodules. The most common causes of liver cirrhosis in the United States are hepatitis B and C, alcoholic liver disease (or a combination of alcoholic disease and hepatitis C), autoimmune liver inflammation, medications, and various metabolic disorders (including nonalcoholic steatohepatitis). A number of things can suggest liver cirrhosis, including clinical features (e.g., jaundice, spider angiomas, hepatomegaly, splenomegaly, and ascites), abnormal lab values (e.g., elevated ALT and AST, hyponatremia, thrombocytopenia, leucopenia, and neutropenia), and specific histological features. The micrograph image shows alcoholic liver cirrhosis.

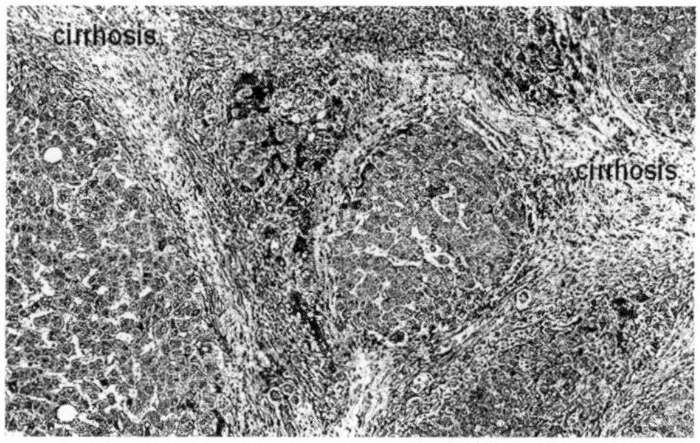

Neoplasms

A neoplasm is an uncoordinated hyperplasia of cells within a tissue. If it persists, it may produce a lump or tumor, which can be benign, premalignant (a confined cancer), or malignant (a metastasized invasive cancer). Neoplasms can be categorized as follows: (1) A dysplasia is the earliest precancerous lesion evident upon biopsy. Low-grade dysplasias rarely become cancerous. (2) A high-grade dysplasia is a carcinoma in situ (CIS) that has not metastasized or invaded surrounding tissues. Basal and squamous cell carcinomas are examples of CIS. The latter has a high risk of metastasizing if left untreated. (3) An invasive carcinoma is one that has a high likelihood of invading surrounding tissues, metastasizing, and spreading via the blood to invade distant organs and tissues. Such cancers are typically lethal if not successfully halted. The image below shows a malignant and highly invasive colorectal carcinoma in a human.

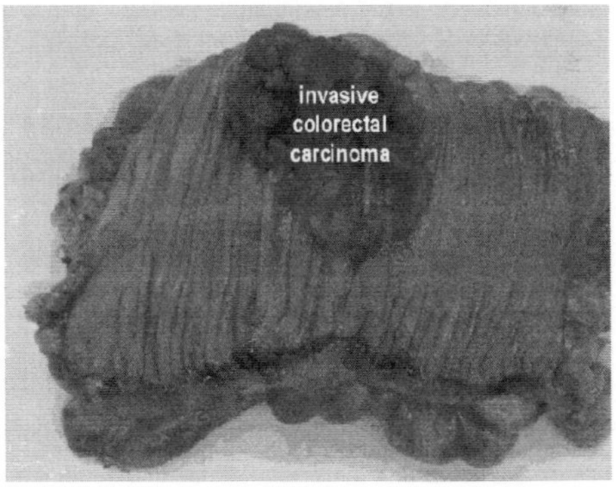

Prostate Biopsies

Prostate biopsies were traditionally performed on men over age 50 whose PSA levels exceeded a certain value. However, several large scale studies have shown conflicting results as to whether this practice is beneficial. Fifteen percent of men in one study with PSA levels of less than 4.0 ng/mL had high-grade prostate cancer, while 65 to 75 percent of men with PSA levels between 4.1 and 9.9 ng/mL were cancer free. The frequency of serious complications due to prostate biopsies is high, and increases with repeated procedures. The presence of blood in the urine, stool, and ejaculate (which can sometimes persist for months); permanent impotence; urinary and/or fecal incontinence; and/or the need for indwelling catheterization to make urination possible may result. Prostate biopsies themselves often cause elevated PSA levels, resulting in a vicious cycle of testing and biopsies. Recent evidence has shown that even in cases where cancer is detected, treatment causes more morbidity and death compared to cases where the cancer was not diagnosed or treated. Patients and their physicians need to make individual decisions about biopsies based on the risks and benefits. The current recommendation is not to screen for prostate cancer in men over 75.

Distinguishing Normal Prostate Tissue from Prostatic Adenocarcinoma

Many early stage prostate carcinomas comprise less than 5 percent of 18-gauge needle biopsy cores, which may also fragment. This issue is further confounded by difficulties visualizing infiltrative alterations in prostate gland architecture associated with variability in histological features. This variability may be due to differences in fixation, sectioning, and staining. Important reference characteristics include the arrangement and nuclear appearance of the basal and luminal cells of the benign glands. Malignant invasive acini may appear to only be embedded within the stroma, and do not elicit the obvious inflammatory reactions seen in other invasive cancers. The micrograph image compares benign and invaded glands (Gleason stage 3).

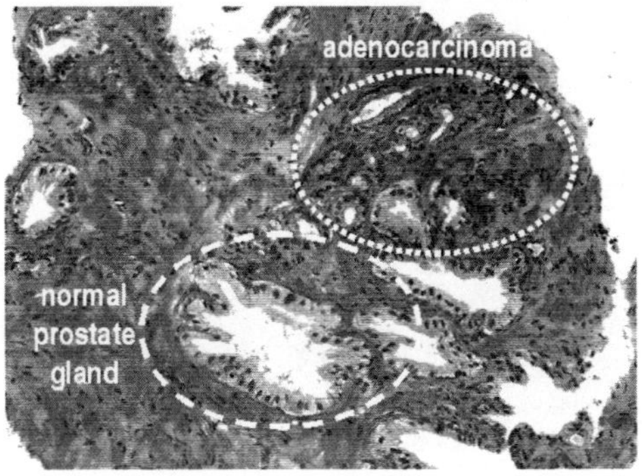

Gleason Stages of Prostate Cancer

A Gleason score for prostate cancer is based on its histological presentation. Cancers with higher Gleason scores are more aggressive, and are associated with a worse prognosis. Small, closely packed cells are associated with cancers with lower Gleason scores. Cellular architecture becomes more diffuse and ill-defined as the cancer progresses.

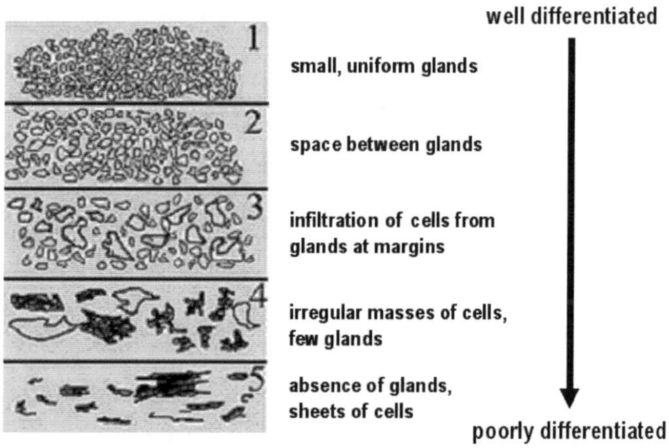

Nondisjunction Events and Trisomies

A nondisjunction event during meiosis can result in a full trisomy, which is when there is an extra copy of an autosome or a sex chromosome. A partial trisomy usually involves a Robertsonian translocation of an extra portion of a chromosome during crossover events, which is when the participating homologous chromosomes break at their centromeres. The long and short arms of each chromosome fuse to form single chromosomes. The fused short chromosome has nonessential genes, and is lost within a few postzygotic mitotic divisions. Trisomies can be classified as both a polysomy (an extra chromosome) and an aneuploidy (an abnormal number of chromosomes compared to the normal karyotype). Most trisomies result in miscarriage, but some affected individuals survive into adulthood with varying degrees of mental and/or physical handicaps. The most common types of trisomies are trisomy 21 (Down syndrome), trisomy 18 (Edwards syndrome), trisomy 13 (Patau syndrome), and two nondisjunctions involving the sex chromosomes: XXX (47,XXX karyotype, or triple X females) and XXY (47,XXY, or Klinefelter syndrome, which affects males). Even a nondisjunction during postzygotic mitosis in early embryogenesis can produce 46,XY/47,XYY mosaics.

Down Syndrome

Down syndrome is caused by whole trisomy 21 or extra copies of portions of chromosome 21 resulting from Robertsonian translocation. This syndrome can affect individuals in a wide variety of ways. Persons with Down syndrome usually exhibit mild to moderate (and occasionally severe) cognitive retardation. They have IQs of around 50, while the average IQ score for the general population is 100. Physical manifestations include microgenia, macroglossia, an epicanthic fold and upward slanting palpebral fissures, a single transverse palmar crease, a gap between the hallux and second toe, and poor muscle tone. Individuals with Down syndrome have a higher risk of congenital heart defects, gastrointestinal reflux disease (GERD), recurrent acute otitis media, thyroid dysfunctions, and obesity. If one or both parents are older at the time of conception, the risk of having a baby with Down syndrome is increased. Amniocentesis and karyotyping are often performed during the 15th to 20th week of pregnancy to determine whether the baby will have Down syndrome.

Klinefelter Syndrome Karyotype

Klinefelter syndrome (47,XXY) is the most common sex chromosome aneuploidy affecting males. The main phenotypic manifestations are hypogonadism and diminished fertility. Other effects are possible, which vary in terms of their degree of severity. They include reduced facial hair and muscle mass; gynecomastia; abnormal body proportions; and speech, learning and personality defects that become more pronounced after the onset of puberty. Many Klinefelter males show no obvious signs. In 47,XYY syndrome, males have an extra Y chromosome. They are often unusually tall and produce extra testosterone, but usually lead normal lives.

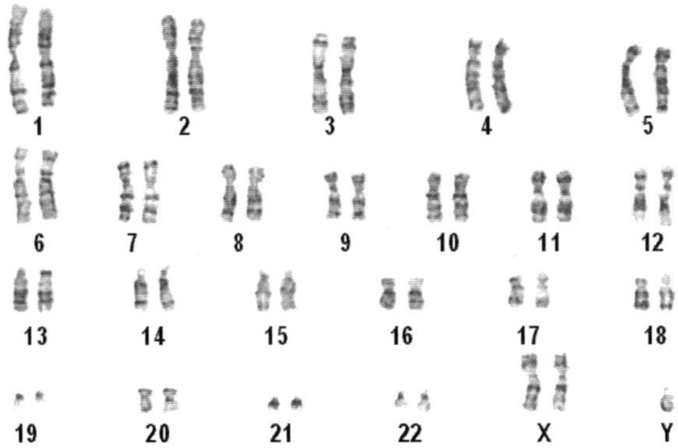

Turner Syndrome Karyotype

Turner syndrome (45 X0) refers to several human female states in which one of the X chromosomes is partially or entirely missing. The most common presentation is monosomy X, which is characterized by a complete absence of the Barr body. Phenotypic expressions include a variety of developmental and medical conditions, especially short stature, failure to start puberty, gonadal dysfunction and amenorrhea, heart defects, and cognitive impairments. This is the only monosomy that is not invariably lethal.

Review Video: Turner Syndrome
Visit mometrix.com/academy and enter code: 802369

Inborn Errors of Metabolism

Most inborn (congenital, or inherited) errors of metabolism are due to defects in a single gene that codes for a specific enzyme. This can result in reduced levels of an essential compound or, conversely, the accumulation of toxic substances or metabolites, the generation of reactive oxygen species and inflammatory cytokines, and/or the activation of various growth factors and other pathogenic factors. Most of the more than 200 congenital metabolic disorders known are due to autosomal recessive alleles. Their overt phenotypic expression is therefore rare. Polygenic congenital disorders are caused by several different genes acting alone or in concert. Their phenotypic expression varies widely depending on the combinations of defective genes that are inherited. These disorders also tend to be multifactorial, and can have either Mendelian (discontinuous) or Galtonian (continuous) distributions within families. The overt expression of disease is moderated or exacerbated by both genetic and environmental/lifestyle factors. X-linked recessive traits are overtly manifested in all heterogametic (XY) individuals (males), but only appear in homogametic (XX) individuals (females) that are homozygous for the trait.

Autosomal Recessive Congenital Metabolic Disorders

Autosomal recessive traits and diseases are only expressed in individuals who are heterozygous for the condition, which means that both parents were/are either heterozygous carriers or homozygous. If two parents are heterozygous, each of their offspring will have a 25 percent chance of having the disorder. Their unaffected children will be heterozygous carriers of the allele. Examples include Tay-Sachs disease, a specific form of polycystic kidney disease, sickle cell train and sickle cell anemia, and the β-thalassemias.

Autosomal Dominant Disorders

Autosomal dominant disorders and disease states appear when a single disease-associated allele is passed on to a carrier's offspring. Rarely, an individual with an autosomal dominant allele will not express the disease or trait due to incomplete or poor penetrance. Dominant diseases rarely skip generations since all individuals who are homozygous or heterozygous for the allele associated with a disease will express the disease. Occasionally, an autosomal dominant disease will appear de novo in a previously unaffected family due to a spontaneous genetic mutation. Examples of autosomal dominant diseases include familial hypercholesterolemia, a specific form of polycystic kidney disease, neurofibromatosis type 1, Marfan syndrome, and Huntington's disease.

Polygenic Diseases

Polygenic diseases are also multifactorial, and involve complex interactions between multiple genes and environmental and/or lifestyle factors. Polygenic traits may be controlled by many genes (each of which has a small effect) or a few genes (each of which has a large effect). Multifactorial diseases aggregate within families, but exhibit continuous (Galtonian) rather than classical discontinuous (Mendelian) inheritance patterns. This is also reflected in monozygotic and dizygotic twin concordance data. These diseases tend to occur more often in one sex than the other, but are not sex-linked, and are often more frequently expressed in specific ethnic or racial groups. Environmental and/or lifestyle factors acting upon variable individual genetic substrates play a major role in the overt expression of multifactorial traits and diseases. Examples include asthma, multiple sclerosis and other autoimmune diseases, many cancers, diabetes mellitus, hypertension, coronary artery disease, the various mood disorders, obesity, alcoholism, and inflammatory bowel disease.

Sex-Linked Disorders

Sex-linked diseases are due to mutations of genes on the X chromosome. Most sex-liked genes are recessive, and dominant sex-linked disorders are very rare. If the father carries a dominant X-link mutation, all of his daughters (XX) and none of his sons (XY) will manifest the disease. If the mother carries the allele, half of all the parents' offspring will have the disease. X-linked recessive diseases are much more common, and are expressed in hemizygous males and homozygous females. Males have no corresponding gene on the Y chromosome, and the trait is expressed if there is a single copy of the allele. Common X-linked recessive diseases include the more common hemophilia A (factor VIII deficiency) and hemophilia B (factor IX deficiency), both of which are due to a recessive allele on the X chromosome. Hemophilia C (factor XI deficiency) is an autosomal disease (chromosome 4) with incomplete penetrance that affects both sexes equally. Its occurrence is largely restricted to Ashkenazi Jews. Two rare examples of X-linked dominant mutations are hypophosphatemic rickets and Rett's syndrome.

Development of Diabetes Mellitus

At least 10 genes are known to be involved in the development of type 2 diabetes (noninsulin-dependent diabetes mellitus). Racial groups in the United States with a high prevalence of diabetes include blacks, Hispanics, and American Indians. Environmental factors, diet, a sedentary lifestyle, and certain medications (e.g., statins used to control cholesterol levels) are important precipitating cofactors. Hypertension, hypercholesterolemia, and obesity are also associated with an increased risk of developing diabetes, but it is unclear whether these associations are causal or consequential, or perhaps both. Type 2 diabetes involves peripheral resistance to insulin, which may be produced at near normal levels. In contrast, type 1 (insulin-dependent) diabetes is an autoimmune disease associated with impaired insulin production. Genes that are known to make people more susceptible to diabetes include several genes of the HLA complex on chromosome 6. Viral infections, including Coxsackie, rubella, measles, mumps, and Epstein-Barr virus; certain medications; high dietary omega-6 to omega-3 fatty acid ratios; and nitrosamines are directly toxic to pancreatic beta cells, and may precipitate an autoimmune overreaction.

Review Video: Diet, Exercise, and Medications for Diabetes
Visit mometrix.com/academy and enter code: 774388

Epigenetic Factors in the Expression of Single Gene and Polygenic Diseases

Epigenetic changes are heritable modifications to the phenotypic expression of genes that do not involve changes (i.e. mutations) to the DNA sequence itself. Methylation of cytosine to 5-methylcytosine in the CpG islands of the promoter regions of genes can switch genes off and inhibit the production of their proteins. Other epigenetic changes involve histone acetylation and chromatin remodeling. Accumulating evidence implicates epigenetic changes in many multifactorial human diseases, including cardiovascular disease, type 2 diabetes mellitus, obesity, and a variety of neurodevelopmental disorders. These changes can be brought about by a variety of environmental factors, such as toxic insults due to heavy metals, pesticides, cigarette smoke, deficiencies in certain vitamins, and low-level ionizing radiation. These changes persist through all subsequent cell divisions in the individual organism, and are passed on to the offspring through multiple generations.

Epigenetic Factors Involved in Cancer

Tumor suppressor genes protect cells from undergoing malignant transformation. They protect the genome from mutagenic events, impede the progression of dysregulated cell cycles, induce apoptosis in cells that have evaded normal cell cycle control mechanisms, and inhibit cell migration and metastasis. Paternally expressed genes stimulate growth and promote oncogenesis, while maternally expressed genes inhibit growth and cancer development. Hypomethylation across the genome can activate nearby oncogenes, while hypermethylation in the CpG promoter regions silences tumor suppressor genes. The *IGF2* gene codes for insulin-like growth factor 2, which promotes cell growth and proliferation. Though highly active during fetal development, it is much less active in the adult body. In adults, only the paternal *IGF2* gene is active; the maternal gene is normally imprinted (switched off). In a number of cancers, the maternal *IGF2* gene is also switched on (loss of imprinting, or LOI), leading to the growth of cancerous cells and the inhibition of apoptosis of damaged cells.

Congenital Disorders

Congenital disorders are conditions arising during development that are present at birth. In addition to the genetic and chromosomal abnormalities already discussed, they include intrauterine problems, infections, defects in morphogenesis and/or organogenesis, maternal diet and toxic insult (e.g., alcohol) during gestation, and even maternal and paternal age and diet prior to conception. Substances that produce birth defects are referred to as teratogens. Common nongenetic congenital defects include fetal alcohol syndrome, patent foramen ovale and/or ductus arteriosus, cleft lip/palate, cryptorchidism, spina bifida, anencephaly, microcephaly, polydactyly, club foot, hypoglossia, and many other conditions. An increasing number of babies are born with infectious diseases and/or drug-related syndromes acquired *in utero*.

Hypersensitivity to Antivenom

Antivenoms (antivenins) are produced by injecting the venom of a snake (or a group of closely related snakes, such as rattlesnakes), an insect, or an arachnid into a horse or other ungulate. The injected animal produces antibodies to the venom, which are then used to treat human envenomation victims. Monovalent antivenoms work against the venom of a single venomous species; polyvalent antivenoms are effective against the venom of a range of species. For example, Aracmyn is effective against the venom of all species of *Latrodectus* (widow spiders) and *Loxosceles* (recluse spiders), and CroFab is effective against the venom of all North American pit vipers. Patients who are sensitive to antivenom components or to horse serum can develop life-threatening anaphylaxis. It is thus critical that a skin sensitivity test be performed prior to IV or IM antivenom administration, and that proper measures be taken if a sensitivity exists.

Incidence of Serious and Fatal Allergic Reactions

Insect envenomations kill about 40 persons annually in the United States. These deaths are due to anaphylaxis caused by insect envenomations. Fifteen percent of adults experience localized allergic reactions to bee and wasp venoms, and three percent of adults and one percent of children experience systemic reactions. Penicillin kills another 400, food allergies cause 150 deaths, and latex causes an estimated 220 cases of anaphylaxis and 3 deaths each year. Three million Americans (1.1 percent of the population) have allergic reactions to peanuts and/or walnuts. Ten million Americans (around three percent of the population) suffer from asthma, and this percentage is higher for the black population. About a quarter of the US population has a strong allergic reaction to urushiol-induced contact dermatitis. Urushiol, produced by all parts of *Toxicodendron* spp. (poison ivy, poison oak, and poison sumac), reacts with membrane proteins on the exposed skin of susceptible persons, eliciting a cellular immune response that causes hives, itchiness, blisters, and vesicles.

Immunologic Deficiencies

Immunologic deficiencies can arise from a failure anywhere in the cascade of interactions between lymphocytes and immunoglobulins. Immunodeficiencies are conditions in which the body's ability to fight infections is diminished or nonexistent. These states can either be inherited or secondarily acquired. Immunodeficiency syndromes can affect humoral immunity (depression/complete suppression of B cells, plasma cells, and/or antibody production) and cellular immunity (depression/complete suppression of T cells and/or granulocytes). They can also result in asplenia and/or impaired complement function. Immunosuppressive therapy used to treat cancer or prevent organ transplant rejection along with infection by Epstein-Barr virus (infectious mononucleosis) or HIV are major causes of secondary immunodeficiency states.

Environmentally Caused Human Diseases

Environmental pollution by toxic anthropogenic compounds that results in direct exposure to and/or ingestion of contaminated foods is a major source of human morbidity and mortality. Methylmercury and polychlorinated biphenyl contamination of otherwise healthy food fishes have led to recommendations regarding maximum consumption of these fishes. The overuse of insecticides, hormones, and antibiotics in the production of crops, meat, and dairy products has also caused widespread and well-publicized adverse health effects. Many people are switching to organically grown crops, free-range poultry, and grass-fed beef as a result. Even more insidious is the nearly ubiquitous presence of transgenically modified (GM) contaminants in conventionally raised crops and grain-fed poultry and livestock. It is now known that potentially toxic GM herbicides (glyphosate and glufosinate) accumulate in the plasma of nonpregnant women. Additionally, a potent transgenic *Bacillus thuringiensis* insecticide (Cry1Ab) and a metabolite of glufosinate have been found in both maternal and fetal blood. Nearly all conventionally raised corn, soy, and canola have been genetically modified, and are exposed to the GM herbicides and insecticides discussed above.

Role of Chiropractic in Treating Back and Neck Pain

Earlier studies focusing on the efficacy and safety of chiropractic manipulation were poorly designed and poorly controlled. An increasing body of recent evidence shows that spinal manipulation is at least as effective and as safe as (and may be safer than repeated epidural steroid injections) conventional nonsurgical methods to treat back and/or neck pain due to scoliosis, lordosis/kyphosis, herniated disks, spondylolisthesis, osteoarthritis, and other common conditions. Chiropractic manipulation performed by properly trained practitioners has not been found to be associated with either the development or exacerbation of cauda equina syndrome.

Osteoporosis

Bone remodeling occurs throughout life. Old bone is continually resorbed and new bone laid down in its place, which results in a dynamic equilibrium. Osteoclasts and osteoblasts dissolve old bone and lay down new bone, respectively. The complex signaling pathways that coordinate these two actions involve parathyroid hormone (PTH) from the parathyroid glands, a growth hormone, interleukin-6 (IL-6), steroid hormones, vitamin D3, and calcitonin from the thyroid gland. Parathyroid hormone from the parathyroid glands increases the plasma concentration of Ca^{2+} by dissolving it from bone; calcitonin removes Ca^{2+} from the blood and lays it down into new bone. PTH stimulates both osteoclasts and osteoblasts, which interact via negative feedback pathways to destroy and lay down bone. Imbalances between these two processes can result in osteopenia and osteoporosis in later years, as more bone is resorbed than deposited. This leads to a progressive reduction in bone density and a thinner, more porous bone structure, which makes bones more prone to fractures.

Giant Cell Tumor of the Bone

Giant cell tumor of the bone is an uncommon type of tumor that is characterized by giant multinucleated cells. It accounts for between 5 and 9 percent of all primary bone tumors (20 percent in China). It is especially common in adults between the ages of 25 and 40, is more common in females, and occurs most commonly in the epiphyseal-metaphyseal region of long bones. Although generally benign, it metastasizes to the lung in about five percent of cases. Image A shows a giant cell bone tumor in the head of the fourth metacarpal of the left hand; image B is a high-magnification micrograph image showing the multinucleated giant cells that are characteristic of this disease.

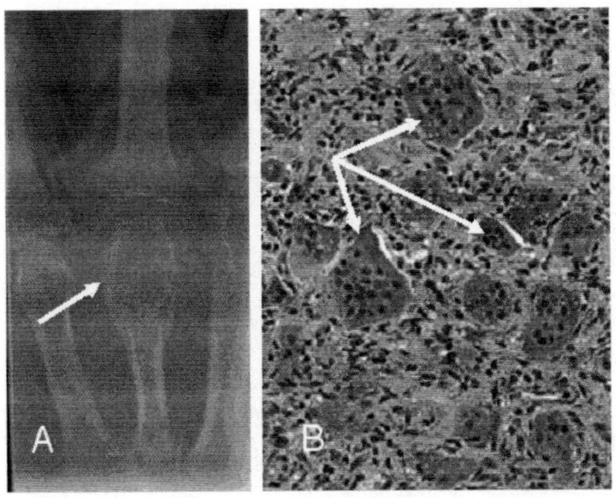

Osteoarthritis

Osteoarthritis affects more than 20 million Americans. It results from a reduction in proteoglycan content and the consequent dehydration of articular cartilages. This leads to inflammatory and degenerative changes in the subchondral bone and synovial capsule. It mainly involves the weight-bearing joints, but the interphalangeal joints of the hands are also commonly affected. Primary osteoarthritis (shown in image) is a poorly understood, progressive, multifactorial disease associated with aging. Secondary osteoarthritis results from previous traumatic injury or another type of insult, and is seen in relatively young people. The X-ray image of left knee osteoarthritis shows extreme narrowing of the joint space (white arrow), the absence of a meniscus, and increased subchondral bone density (black arrows).

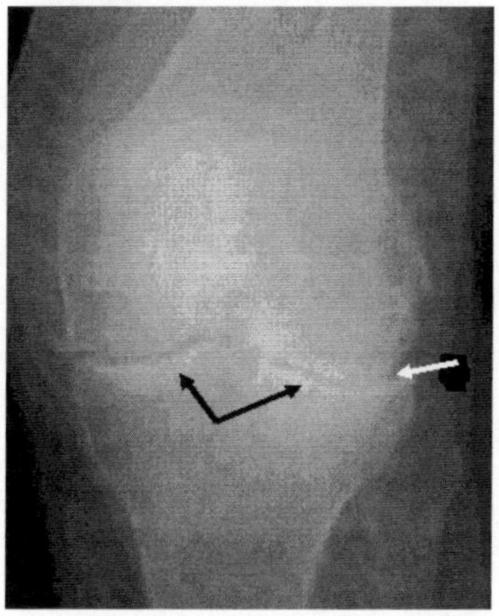

Scoliosis

Scoliosis refers to abnormal lateral bending of the spine. It may be present at birth (congenital scoliosis), or it may first appear during childhood, adolescence, or adult life. Idiopathic scoliosis due to unknown but presumably multifactorial (including genetic) cause(s) is the most common form, accounting for 65 percent of all cases. Congenital scoliosis accounts for 15 percent of cases, and 10 percent of cases are secondary to an underlying traumatic collapse due to injury, a neuromuscular disease, or another type of disease. The X-ray image shows thoracic dextroscoliosis and lumbar levoscoliosis.

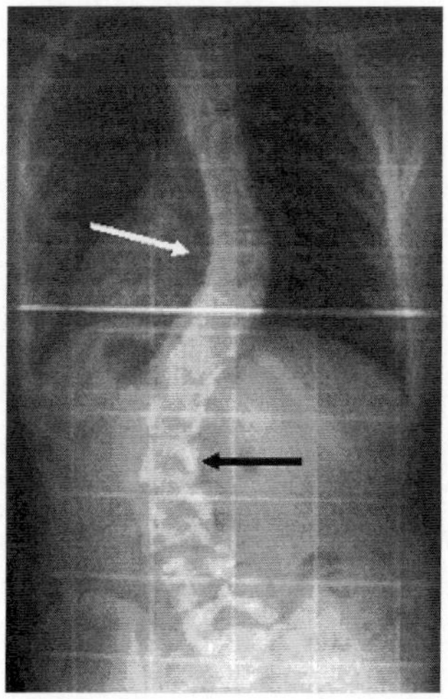

Spondylolisthesis

Spondylolisthesis is the forward slippage of one vertebra (and the spinal column above it) over the one beneath. It most commonly occurs in the lumbar-sacral region. It is graded according to how much of the vertebral body (centrum) has slipped: grade 1 = 25 percent slippage, grade 2 = 50 percent slippage, grade 3 = 75 percent slippage, and grade 4 = 100 percent slippage. Spondyloptosis is when the entire vertebral body has fallen off the spine beneath. Spondylolisthesis can be asymptomatic, or it can produce symptoms that range from lower back pain to stiffness in the muscles of the buttocks and thighs, nerve damage, and sciatica. The X-ray image of the lateral lumbar spine shows a spondylolisthesis at L5-S1.

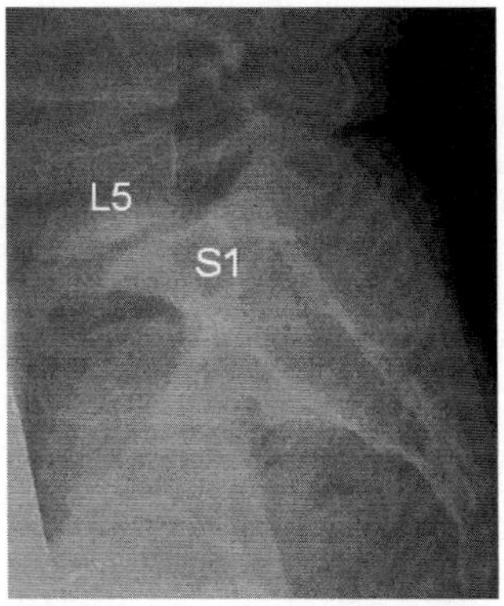

Normal and Stenosed Spinal Canals and Disc Herniation

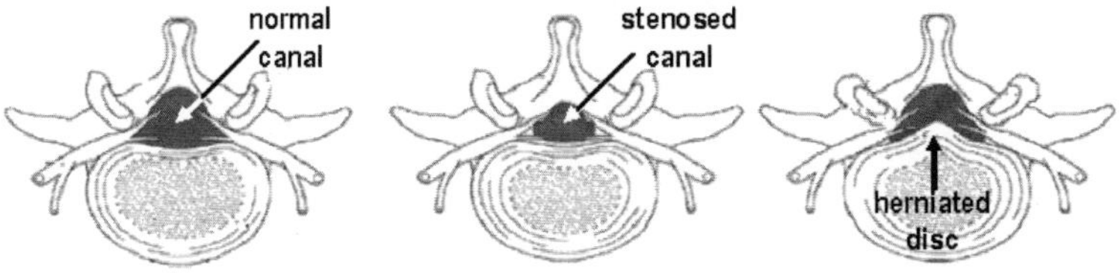

Spinal Stenosis

Spinal stenosis can result from spinal osteoarthritis, degenerative diseases of the spine (e.g., Paget's disease and achondroplasia), congenital spinal defects, a herniated disk and/or scarring resulting from its surgical reduction, traumatic injury, or spinal tumor. Symptoms can be progressive, and include unilateral or bilateral radiculopathies, muscular weakness in the lower limb(s), claudication, ataxia, impotence, and urinary and/or bowel incontinence. Treatment options include chiropractic adjustments, physical therapy and specific exercises, massage and/or acupuncture, alternating hot and cold packs, and medication (including pain medication when necessary).

Scapholunate Advanced Collapse (SLAC) Wrist

SLAC (scapholunate advanced collapse) wrist is the most common form of osteoarthritis of the wrist, and results in scapholunate dissociation and scaphoid rotation, loss of joint space, and carpal collapse. This is shown in the radiograph image (© Dr. William H. Light, used with permission). Associated pain is moderate to severe depending on disease progression. Treatment with NSAIDs, acetaminophen, and/or opioids may be indicated; long-term treatment with NSAIDs and acetaminophen is associated with renal failure, and a proportion of patients are liable to abuse opioids. Treatment options for severe SLAC are surgical, and all of them have serious adverse effects. An SLAC reconstruction involves scaphoid excision and arthrodesis of the capitate, the lunate, the hamate, and the triquetrum. Proximal row carpectomy (PRC) involves resecting the proximal row of carpals to allow for articulation of the capitate within the lunate fossa. Failure of either procedure will necessitate salvage wrist arthrodesis (fusion).

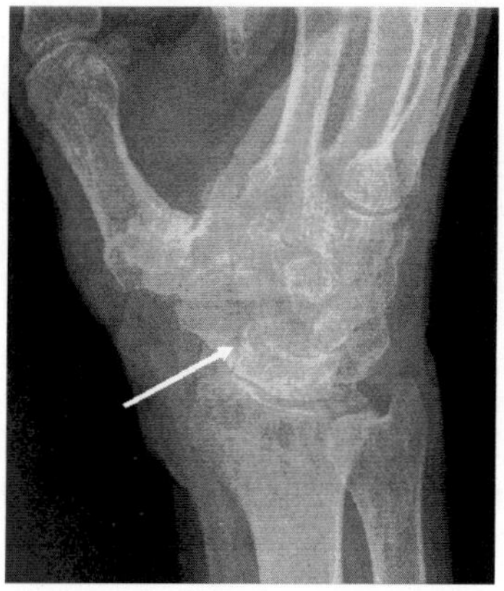

Degenerative Joint Disease

Degenerative joint disease involves excessive wear and tear of articular cartilage, usually with osteophyte growth and an increase in the density of the subchondral bone, which result from increased pressure on the bone and stenosis of the joint space. Degenerative joint disease may or may not involve inflammation of the bursa and accompanying tendonitis. Rheumatoid arthritis is a much rarer autoimmune disease affecting one percent of the human population, with women affected more often than men. It erodes the cartilage and joint lining, resulting in painful synovial hyperplasia and swelling, fibrosis and ankylosis, and eventual bone erosion and crippling deformities of the joints. Unlike osteoarthritis, rheumatoid arthritis can cause major systemic problems.

Acute Gouty Arthritis

Acute gouty arthritis is due to hyperuricemia. It occurs when elevated serum urate levels precipitate out as crystals in synovial joint fluid, which leads to acute attacks involving very painful inflammation, erythema, and swelling. The most common site of inflammation is the metatarsal-phalangeal joint and surrounding tissues of the big toe, but attacks can also occur at other sites. Uric acid can also form tophi in joints, cartilage, and bones anywhere in the body; precipitate as kidney stones; and even cause renal impairment. Hyperuricemia can result from dietary intake and/or genetic predisposition that causes an overproduction of uric acid or renal impairment. The latter results in underexcretion of monosodium urate (this is responsible for nearly 90 percent of all gout attacks). Diuretics taken to control blood pressure can also cause hyperuricemia.

Skeletal Muscle Diseases

Muscle diseases can have multiple and in some cases unknown causes. Myopathies are skeletal muscle diseases that are not caused by an underlying neuropathy. They are often degenerative, but can be due to drug side effects (e.g., statins), toxic insult, cancer, virus infection, or an autoimmune disorder. Myositis refers to several inflammatory and frequently degenerative myopathies: polymyositis, dermatomyositis, and inclusion body myositis. Fibromyalgia is likely due to genetic causes, and more frequently affects young to middle-aged women. Muscular dystrophy is another genetic disease. The presenting features are muscle weakening and wasting away. Muscle tissue is replaced by fatty deposits. Rhabdomyolysis is a potentially life-threatening condition involving muscle tissue breakdown and the release of myoglobin into the blood, which can clog and damage the kidneys. Statin medications, crush injuries, and severe burns are some precipitating causes of rhabdomyolysis. Denervation resulting from a herniated disk and peripheral neuropathy can also produce muscle weakness and atrophy.

ALS

Amyotrophic lateral sclerosis (ALS), more commonly called Lou Gehrig's disease, involves the progressive degeneration of the motor neurons in the ventral horns of the spinal cord and the motor cortex. ALS can also affect other cortical neurons. Half of all patients exhibit mild cognitive and other behavioral changes, and 5 to 15 percent suffer frank dementia. Many, however, show no cognitive impairment. ALS is a fatal neurodegenerative disease involving progressive weakness, muscle atrophy, spasticity and fasciculations, dysarthria, and dysphagia that leads to a total inability to speak. Most patients die within two to five years from respiratory compromise or pneumonia, but some patients may live for many years. A notable example is the still living, though completely paralyzed and unable to speak, prominent theoretical physicist Dr. Steven Hawking, whose disease first appeared in 1962.

Review Video: Amyotrophic Lateral Sclerosis (ALS)
Visit mometrix.com/academy and enter code: 178603

Compartment Syndrome

Compartment syndrome is a limb- and life-threatening condition resulting from decreased perfusion and ischemia due to elevated intracompartmental pressure. Rapid fasciotomy to relieve pressure is required when subfascial pressures exceed 30 mm Hg. This condition can result from fractures to the forearm or leg, severe hematoma, hemorrhage, prolonged elevation of the lower legs following trauma or surgery, deep vein thrombosis (DVT), crush injuries and burns, and envenomation by viperine or crotaline snakes (Old World vipers and pit vipers, respectively). Fasciotomy performed within six hours of ischemic compromise results in almost total recovery of limb function, which is the upper limit for limb viability. Excessive use of creatine supplements by athletes and body builders and extreme exercise (e.g., marathon running) have also been implicated as a cause of compartment syndrome.

Chronic Alcoholic Myopathy

Chronic alcoholic myopathy occurs in half of alcohol abusers, who present with ataxia, myalgia, cramps, selective atrophy of type II fibers (so-called "fast twitch" fibers), and reductions in total body muscle mass that are as high as 30 percent. This is due to both peripheral neuropathologic deficits and direct toxic myopathologic insult from the inhibitory effects of alcohol and metabolite, acetaldehyde, on muscle protein synthesis.

Diabetic Neuropathy

Diabetic neuropathy can involve both the somatic and autonomic nervous systems. It arises from a complex series of microvascular complications caused by chronic hyperglycemia. Elevated plasma glucose activates protein kinase Cβ (PKCβ) by several pathways: (1) excessive flux of glucose through the glycolytic pathway, resulting in abnormal elevations of diacylglycerol (DAG); (2) overproduction of superoxide radicals due to excessive flux of reducing equivalents through the electron transport chain; (3) hypoxia-induced vascular endothelial growth factor (VEGF); (4) activation of the polyol pathway; (5) nonenzymatic glycosylation of certain proteins, resulting in advanced glycation end products (AGEs) such as hemoglobin A1c (HbA1c), which is commonly used to assess glycemic control in diabetics over a three-month period; and (6) overproduction of angiotensin II and endothelin I. Factors 1 through 6 as well as elevated levels of PKCβ lead to angiogenesis and vascular proliferation that give rise to the microvascular complications seen in type 2 diabetic neuropathy, nephropathy, and retinopathy.

Diabetic neuropathy is the leading cause of nontraumatic limb amputations. Loss of sensation due to peripheral nerve damage results in cuts and minor infections being ignored. This, combined with reduced vascularization in the extremities due to atherosclerosis and small vessel disease, often leads to ulceration, tissue necrosis, and gangrene, necessitating progressive amputations. Diabetic neuropathy can also cause Charcot foot, urinary tract infections and incontinence, and sexual dysfunction in both sexes. Diabetic autonomic dysfunction can result in a range of digestive disorders, including gastroparesis, orthostatic hypotension, and failure to recognize medication-induced hypoglycemia, which can have a potentially fatal outcome.

Other Causes of Peripheral Neuropathy

Peripheral neuropathies have many other causes aside from diabetes mellitus. These include alcoholism, autoimmune diseases (e.g., rheumatoid arthritis, lupus, and Guillain-Barré syndrome), exposure to heavy metals and other toxic insults, bacterial (e.g., Lyme disease) or viral infections (e.g., varicella-zoster, hepatitis C, and HIV), inherited diseases (e.g., amyloid polyneuropathy and Charcot-Marie-Tooth disease), trauma or repetitive overuse strain mononeuropathies (e.g., carpal tunnel syndrome), tumors, vitamin deficiencies (e.g., thiamine, pyridoxine, niacin, or methylcobalamin), and underlying thyroid, liver, or kidney disease.

Encephalitis

Encephalitis is a typically life-threatening inflammation of the brain due to infection by a virus, prion, bacterium, or protozoan. Acute viral encephalitis can have many causes, including rabies virus; herpes simplex virus; enteroviruses (e.g., poliovirus and coxsackievirus); rubeola, mumps, and rubella viruses; St. Louis, western equine, and Venezuelan encephalitis viruses; and West Nile virus. Bacterial encephalitis can be caused by a primary or secondary infection due to a disease such as syphilis, or by staph infections resulting from envenomations by recluse spiders of the genus *Loxosceles*. Protozoal brain infections can be due to toxoplasmosis, malaria, or other parasites. Secondary encephalitis rarely occurs as a post-vaccination complication.

Meningitis

Meningitis is an inflammation of the meninges surrounding the brain and spinal cord. Most meningitis results from viral infections, which generally resolve within a week or two. Bacterial meningitis is less common, and is a much more serious and potentially life-threatening illness. Secondary bacterial meningitis commonly results from upper respiratory, sinus, or ear infections by *Neisseria meningitidis*, *Streptococcus pneumoniae*, or *Haemophilus influenzae*. Chronic meningitis can be caused by fungal pathogens, but is quite rare. Those presenting with meningitis typically exhibit the following symptoms: headache, neck stiffness, high fever, confusion and altered sensorium, photophobia, and/or phonophobia. In addition to death, complications in children can include deafness, blindness, epilepsy, aphasia, memory loss, cognitive deficits, and paralysis.

Review Video: Meningitis
Visit mometrix.com/academy and enter code: 277418

Arachnoid Cysts

Arachnoid cysts form when the two lipid layers of the arachnoid separate and become filled with cerebrospinal fluid. Primary (congenital) arachnoid cysts result from developmental abnormalities, and are present at birth. Secondary (acquired) arachnoid cysts result from head trauma, meningitis, tumors, or brain surgery complications. Most form around the temporal lobe. Cysts usually develop in infancy, but can develop up through young adulthood. Females are four times more likely to develop these lesions than males. The MRI image shows a 25-year-old woman with a left frontotemporal arachnoid cyst.

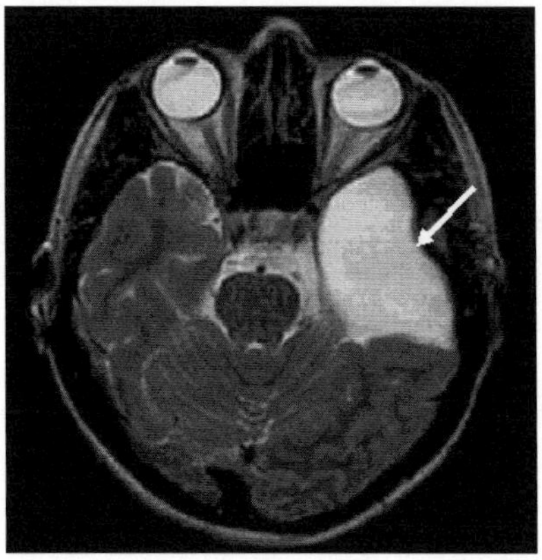

Huntington's Disease

Huntington's disease is a progressive and ultimately fatal neurodegenerative disease due to an autosomal dominant mutation on chromosome 4. This mutation causes a CAG repeat—a repetitive sequence of the nucleobases cytosine, adenine, and guanine—to occur more often than normal. The number of repeats increases with each generation, resulting in Huntington's disease appearing at earlier ages. It usually appears in the third or fourth decade of life. Neuronal degeneration can occur anywhere in the brain, but is especially common in the striatum, where it causes progressively worsening stereotypical choreiform movements. Behavioral and cognitive changes include hallucinations and paranoia, irritability, memory loss, confusion, and personality changes.

Alzheimer's Disease

Age-associated dementias affect some 24 million people over the age of 65 worldwide. Alzheimer's disease accounts for more than 75 percent of age-associated dementia cases. Other causes include frontotemporal dementia and vascular dementia. Dementia is characterized by progressive deterioration in all cognitive and memory functions and behavioral changes. The disease progresses over a period of 7 to 10 years, after which point the patient is in a chronic vegetative state. The disease is invariably fatal. The disease is characterized by plaques of amyloid peptides between 40 and 42 amino acids in length and neurofibrillary tangles of paired helical aggregations of hyperphosphorylated tau protein. There is an accompanying loss of microtubule stability. These lesions form primarily in the hippocampus and the cortex. The postmortem micrograph image shows senile plaques in the cerebral cortex in a patient with presenile onset Alzheimer's disease. Some evidence suggests that regular caffeine consumption may both protect against and even reverse the mental impairments seen in this devastating disease.

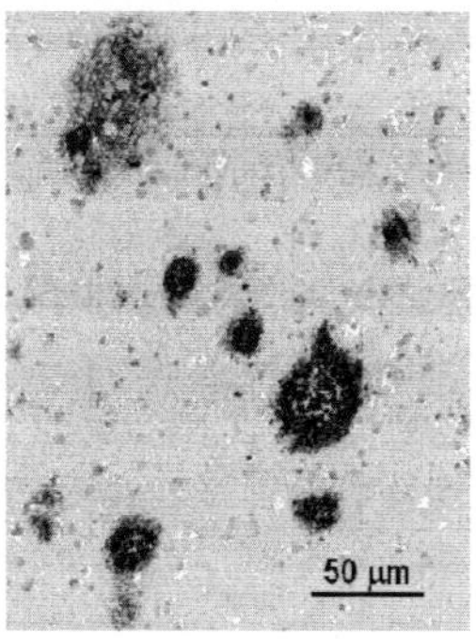

Parkinson's Disease

Parkinson's disease is an idiopathic neurodegenerative syndrome characterized by progressive loss of dopaminergic neurons in the substantia nigra projecting to the striatum (caudate nucleus and putamen) on each side of the diencephalon. The classical physical signs include resting tremor, rigidity, bradykinesia, and ataxia. Later signs may include behavioral changes, cognitive dysfunction, and dementia in advanced cases. Pathologic changes include Lewy bodies, which are abnormal aggregates of alpha-synuclein fibrils. Classical Lewy bodies are cytoplasmic inclusions in the brainstem associated with motor dysfunction; cortical Lewy bodies are associated with cognitive dysfunction, memory loss, and dementia. They are very similar to the lesions that occur with both Lewy body dementia and Alzheimer's disease (they are more commonly associated with the former), both of which may occur along with Parkinson's disease. Secondary Parkinson's may be caused by neuroleptic medications such as the phenothiazines and haloperidol, or by multiple lacunar infarcts. Parkinson's disease affects about 1 percent of those over 60 years of age, and about 4 percent of those over 80 years of age. The micrograph image shows intraneural Lewy bodies in the substantia nigra of a Parkinson's patient.

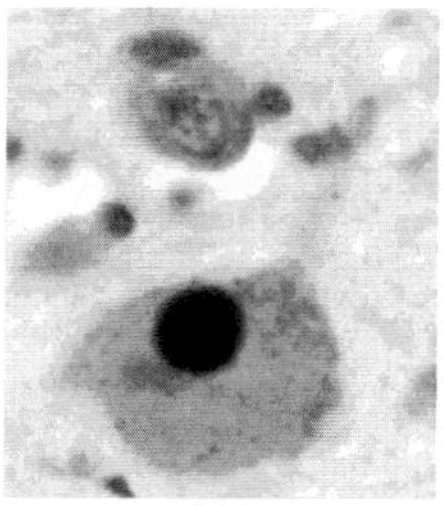

Orthopedic and Chiropractic Subluxation

An orthopedic subluxation refers to a significant structural displacement of a joint, which is usually evident on a radiograph. A chiropractic subluxation, or "nonallopathic lesion," refers to any dysfunctional segment. There may or may not be a significant anatomical displacement. This distinction is acknowledged by the World Health Organization. Traditional chiropractors adhere to the metaphysical and vitalistic notion that one or more vertebral subluxations cause altered "nerve vibrations" that interfere with the body's flow of innate intelligence. However, most present-day chiropractors are "mixers" to one extent or another, and combine the reductionist, evidence-based foundations of science with an integrative and holistic approach to health and well-being. They tend to eschew the use of the controversial term "subluxation." An increasing body of evidenced-based research has shown that chiropractic treatment is an effective and conservative alternative approach to address conditions such as spinal stenosis that offers significant relief in many cases. It also allows patients to avoid the adverse consequences of epidural steroid injections or surgical intervention. As a result, chiropractic and conventional medical approaches are gradually merging into a mutually cooperative venture.

Atherosclerosis

Atherosclerosis is characterized by the thickening of arterial walls due to chronic inflammation and the accumulation of cholesterol and other fatty deposits as plaque. For decades, conventional wisdom has been that elevated levels of low-density lipoproteins (LDL-C) and low levels of high-density lipoproteins (HDL-C) were the major factors underlying this disease. However, many patients suffering from acute MIs have optimal LDL-C levels. The apoB:apo A-1 ratio showing the balance between atherogenic and antiatherogenic particles is emerging as a much more sensitive indicator of MI risk. It is likely more important than total cholesterol, triglycerides, or absolute levels of LDLs and HDLs. The apoB:apo A-1 ratio can also be determined without the need for fasting labs. Emerging evidence increasingly implicates C-reactive protein, inflammatory cytokines, and lowered levels of adiponectin in the pathogenesis of atherosclerosis, rather than serum lipids per se. However, in medicine, as in everything else, old habits and paradigms die hard. Evidence also suggests that excessively low LDL levels may play a role in oncogenesis. This issue is far from settled, however.

Atherosclerotic Lesions on Arteries

Atherogenesis is initiated by the inflammatory accumulation of macrophages onto the vascular endothelium intima, and thence into the subendothelial space. Here, macrophages promote invasion by LDLs and other lipids. These, in turn, initiate platelet and activated monocyte adhesion, along with the release of PDGF, IGF-1, and other growth factors. This leads to smooth muscle proliferation and migration from the tunica media into the endothelium. The tunica intima is grossly expanded from a thickness of one cell (~10 μm) to approximately one-third of a millimeter. The arterial lumen is reduced to about 35 percent of its original diameter.

Risk Factors

In addition to metabolic disorders such as dyslipidemia, the following risk factors are associated with atherosclerosis: diabetes mellitus-induced advanced glycation end products and reactive oxygen species (generated by excess flux through the glycolytic pathway and the electron transport chain), elevated serum homocysteine and C-reactive protein and decreased apo A-1 caused by vitamin B_{12} deficiency or renal impairment due to diabetes and/or hypertension, mechanical shear resulting from hypertension, and exogenous toxins like those found in cigarette smoke (including secondhand smoke). Other risk factors include obesity, alcoholism, genetic factors, sex and age (atherosclerosis is more common in males than pre-menopausal females; after menopause, the risks are similar), and stress.

Cardiomyopathy

Cardiomyopathy refers to any disease that damages the heart muscle. Dilated cardiomyopathy occurs when left or right ventricular contraction is impaired, leading to progressive cardiac remodeling and hypertrophy. It is a significant cause of congestive heart failure. Hypertrophic cardiomyopathy is a generally asymptomatic idiopathic condition where part of the myocardium hypertrophies. This occurs as the sarcomeres increase in size and disrupt the normal alignment of the myocytes. A common feature of this condition is asymmetric septal hypertrophy, and it is a major cause of sudden death in young athletes. In restrictive cardiomyopathy, the walls of the atria and/or ventricles become rigid due to amyloid buildup and fail to fill adequately. This reduces the preload, resulting in inadequate filling of the ventricles. It eventually causes diastolic dysfunction and cardiac failure. The micrograph image shows postmortem cardiomyopathy. (A) shows amyloidosis, and (B) shows fibrosis.

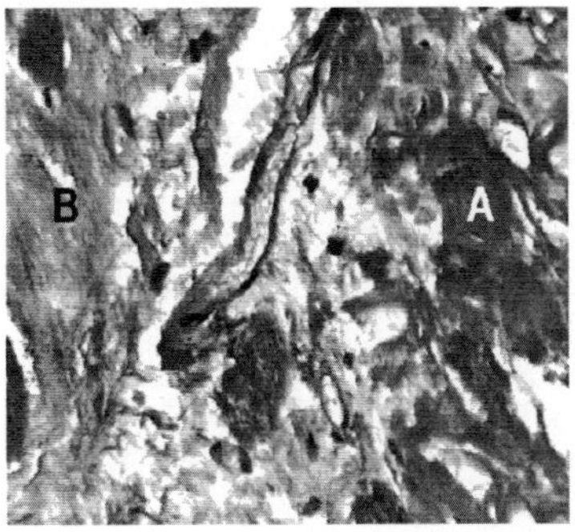

Functional and Structural Gastrointestinal Disorders

Functional GI disorders are those syndromes that have no identifiable organic, structural, physiological, or biochemical cause. They include functional gastritis/GERD, dyspepsia, irritable bowel syndrome (IBS), functional constipation, and functional diarrhea. However, many of these disorders may, like gastric and duodenal ulcers, prove to have an organic basis. Side effects of certain medications can also cause these symptoms. Structural GI disorders are those that can be associated with structural lesions, physiological or biochemical abnormalities, or infectious pathogens. They include gastric and duodenal ulcers, diverticulosis and diverticulitis, colon polyps, ulcerative colitis and Crohn's disease, colorectal cancer, hemorrhoids, perianal abscesses, anal fissures, and anal fistulae.

Peptic Ulcers

The majority of peptic ulcers, previously considered to be functional disturbances related to stress, are now known to result from chronic inflammation in response to infection by *Helicobacter pylori*. This is a helical, gram-negative, flagellated bacterium that resides in the gastric and/or duodenal mucosa of more than 80 percent of infected individuals. Some 60 percent of gastric ulcers and 90 percent of duodenal ulcers appear to be due to *H. pylori*. Nonselective cyclooxygenase inhibitors that prevent the synthesis of COX-1, which protects the gastric mucosa from the corrosive effects of HCl, are another major cause of ulcers. A small percentage are caused by tumors. *Helicobacter pylori* produces an enzyme called urease, which metabolizes the urea normally secreted into the stomach into CO_2 and NH_3. This ammonia is then reduced to NH_4^+ through the acceptance of a proton from the HCl, which neutralizes the acid. In a few individuals, the accumulation of ammonia and other products produced by *H. pylori* can damage the mucosa and initiate a lesion, which can lead to ulcer formation.

Colorectal Carcinoma

Colorectal cancers are complex diseases associated with increasing age, lifestyle, and genetic factors. They involve the epigenetic silencing of tumor suppressor genes. This leads to the activation of oncogenes such as *c-myc* and the hyperexpression of cyclin D1, which drive a progressive transformation from a precancerous adenoma to a malignant carcinoma. Spontaneous mutations of an adenomatous polyposis gene are common events in the development of colorectal cancers. The mutations are inherited in only one percent of cases.

The micrograph image compares a premalignant colorectal polyp (adenoma) with normal mucosal tissue.

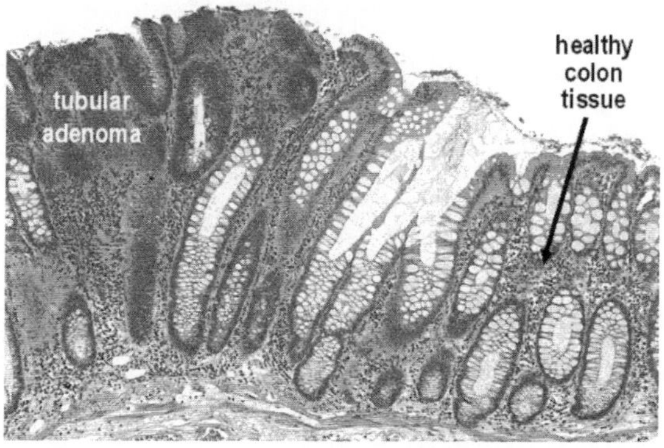

Types of Diabetes

Type 1 diabetes (insulin-dependent diabetes mellitus, or juvenile-onset diabetes) is caused by a failure of the pancreatic beta cells to produce insulin. In type 2 diabetes (NIDDM, or non-insulin-dependent diabetes mellitus), the pancreas produces adequate amounts of insulin, but the peripheral tissues cannot effectively utilize it. Both type 1 and type 2 diabetes are chronic and progressive disorders that often result in a variety of macrovascular atherosclerotic complications, including coronary artery disease, peripheral arterial disease, stroke, and stroke-related dementia. Microvascular complications include diabetic retinopathy, nephropathy, and neuropathy. Gestational diabetes occurs during pregnancy, and the individual usually experiences a postpartum recovery. However, it may portend the subsequent development of type 2 diabetes.

Microvascular Complications of Diabetes Mellitus

The microvascular complications of diabetes mellitus are caused by a complex interaction of multiple abnormal pathways. These include (1) excessive flux of glucose through the glycolytic pathway, resulting in abnormally elevated levels of diacylglycerol; (2) overproduction of superoxide radicals due to excessive flux through the electron transport chain; (3) hypoxia-induced vascular endothelial growth factor (VEGF); (4) activation of the polyol pathway; (5) nonenzymatic glycosylation of certain proteins resulting in advanced glycation end products (AGEs); and (6) overproduction of angiotensin II and endothelin 1. All of these processes generate abnormal levels of protein kinase Cβ (PKCβ1 and PKCβ2), which causes oxidative stress. This, in turn, feeds back into the foregoing processes.

Diabetic Nephropathy

Diabetic nephropathy, a major microvascular complication of diabetes mellitus, is characterized by diffuse nodular glomerulosclerosis and glomerulonephritis, resulting in proteinuria and hypoalbuminemia. The resulting kidney damage leads to a reduced glomerular filtration rate, fluid retention, and edema due to lowered colloid osmotic pressure from protein loss, chronic hypertension, and further renal impairment. Those with end-stage renal disease may require dialysis and/or a kidney transplant. The micrograph image shows nodular glomerulosclerosis, which is seen in diabetic nephropathy. (A) shows the obliteration of glomerular capillary loops by hyaline infiltrate, (B) shows the fibrin cap, and (C) shows the abnormal proliferation of mesangial cells.

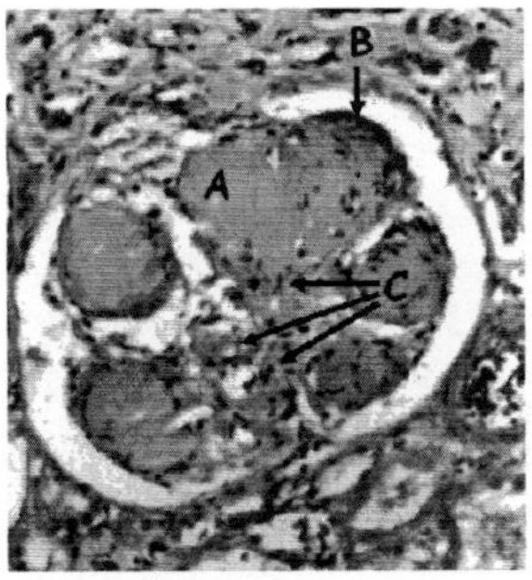

Laboratory Tests for Thyroid Function

Blood tests used to ascertain the presence of thyroid disorders include thyroid-stimulating hormone (TSH), tetraiodothyronine (T4) and triiodothyronine (T3, or thyroxine), thyroglobulin (TG, for papillary or follicular adenocarcinoma), calcitonin (for medullary thyroid cancer), and, less commonly, thyroxine-binding globulin (TBG). A thyroid-releasing hormone (TRH) suppression challenge is sometimes used to evaluate suspected major depressive disorder, bipolar disorder, or cocaine, amphetamine, or PCP abuse.

Urogenital Diseases and Disorders

Congenital urogenital deformities include hypospadias, epispadias, and varicoceles in males, and labial fusion in females. Congenital defects affecting both sexes include renal agenesis, renal hypoplasia, supernumerary kidneys, and ectopic kidney. Congenital urogenital abnormalities can be due to the intrauterine environment, teratogenesis, chromosomal aberration, medication effects, or infection (e.g., syphilis or HIV). Medication side effects, aging processes, and diseases such as hypertension and diabetes mellitus can cause a variety of urogenital problems, including renal impairment, erectile dysfunction and impotence in males, loss of arousal, dyspareunia, and anorgasmia in females. Sexually transmitted infections can cause a variety of symptoms, including painful urination, discharge from the penis or vagina, abdominal or testicular pain, and painful intercourse. Late stage syphilis or AIDS can cause severe medical complications and death.

Prostatitis and Benign Prostatic Hyperplasia

Prostatitis is an inflammation and/or infection of the prostate gland primarily affecting men under age 50. It often results in severe prostatodynia (pain) and changes in urination frequency. Benign prostatic hyperplasia (BPH) is a common, noncancerous prostatic disorder that occurs in most men after age 60, particularly in developed countries. It is characterized by delayed, intermittent, or weak urination; frequent nocturnal urination; urinary urgency and incontinence; and incomplete emptying of the bladder. BPH is treated with alpha blockers and/or 5α-reductase inhibitors, both of which often have adverse sexual side effects.

COPD

Chronic obstructive pulmonary disease (COPD) can refer to either chronic bronchitis or emphysema, although in most cases of COPD the two conditions occur together. Chronic bronchitis is characterized by hyperplasia and hypertrophy of the goblet cells and mucous glands lining the airway, which cause chronic cough and sputum production. Emphysema occurs when the walls of the alveoli are damaged or break down, resulting in fewer and enlarged air sacs. COPD is diagnosed when the FEV1/FVC ratio is below 0.7. Unlike asthma, COPD is not reversible, but it can be managed with rehabilitation, medications and inhalers, supplemental oxygen, and, in some cases, lung transplantation. Smoking is the leading cause of COPD, and causes 80 to 90 percent of all cases. Cessation of smoking is the single most important factor in preventing continued progression of COPD. The micrograph image shows normal alveoli (A) and the disrupted walls and enlarged alveolar sacs that occur with emphysema (B).

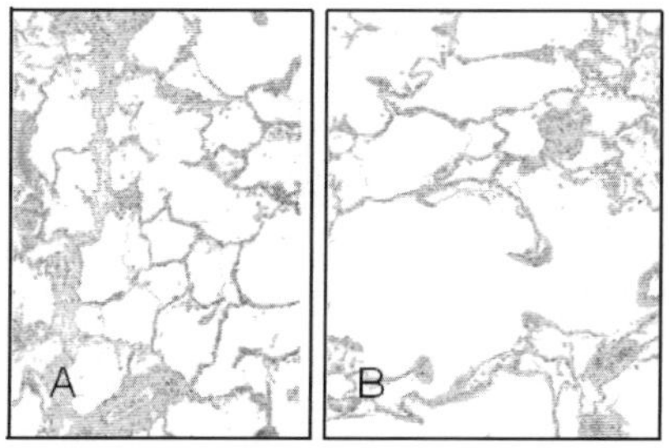

Lung Cancers

Small-cell lung cancer (SCLC) is an aggressive carcinoma that quickly metastasizes and spreads to other tissues in the body, very often the brain, before symptoms become apparent. Non-small-cell lung cancer (NSCLC) refers to any epithelial lung carcinoma other than SCLC. It is the type of lung cancer almost always seen in those who have never smoked. NSCLCs include the following subtypes: squamous cell carcinoma, adenocarcinoma of the lung, large-cell carcinoma, and mixed types. NSCLCs are generally more amenable to surgical resection than SCLCs, but the prognosis for all lung cancers is poor. Lung cancers are almost always caused by smoking or secondhand exposure to tobacco smoke, but a minority of cases are caused by exposure to other environmental or occupational carcinogens, such as radon gas and asbestos or infectious agents. The five-year survival rates for the different types of lung cancers are as follows: SCLC, 5 percent; NSCLCs: squamous cell, 15 percent; adenocarcinoma of the lung, 17 percent; and large-cell carcinoma, 11 percent.

Deep Vein Thrombosis

Venous thromboembolism occurs when an embolism dislodges from a venous thrombus. It manifests in deep vein thrombosis (DVT), the formation of a thrombus in a deep vein, typically in a lower limb, or in the pelvic vein. The primary danger of DVT is the seeding of a clot to the lungs, which can cause a life-threatening pulmonary embolism (PE), which is a blockage of an artery in the lung. The mortality rate for an untreated PE is 26 percent according to the results of a 1960 placebo-controlled clinical trial that was never repeated for ethical reasons. Risk factors for DVT include older age, major or orthopedic surgery, certain cancers, orthopedic immobilization in a cast or a splint, sitting immobilization during long-distance travel by air or automobile, certain medications and chemotherapy, heavy smoking, inborn thrombophilias, recent pregnancy, polycythemia vera, and other factors.

Lymphocytopenia

Lymphocytopenia results from a number of unrelated causes. Among these are infectious diseases caused by bacteria or viruses (especially HIV), autoimmune disorders such as rheumatoid arthritis and lupus, steroid treatment, Hodgkin's disease and other blood disorders, immunosuppressive chemotherapy, anticoagulation therapy, malnutrition, large-dose radiation treatments, certain rare inherited disorders, and severe stress or excessive or prolonged physical exercise that results in the release of cortisol.

Lymphatic Disorders

Some of the most frequently seen lymph disorders include tonsillitis, Hodgkin's lymphoma, lymphadenitis and lymphangitis, various lymphedemas, lymphadenopathy syndrome, lymphogranuloma venereum, and the lymphomas. The lymphatic system is a common avenue for metastasizing cancers. Elephantiasis results from lymphatic blockage due to infection by certain tropical microfilaria (e.g., *Wuchereria bancrofti* and *Brugia* spp.), which are transmitted through mosquito bites. It often manifests as grotesque swelling of the legs and scrotum and thickening of the skin. A non-infectious form of elephantiasis called podoconiosis is prevalent in the volcanic highland zones of East Africa, Central and South America, northwest India, and Sri Lanka. It is due to the absorption of silica particles from the soil into the bare feet of agrarian workers. Unlike filarial elephantiasis, the thigh is rarely involved.

Primary and Secondary Hemochromatosis

Primary hemochromatosis is an inherited autosomal recessive disorder that causes excessive intestinal iron absorption, resulting in toxic levels of iron accumulating in the body. This can cause organ failure in midlife, particularly failure of the liver, pancreas, and heart. This can lead to liver cirrhosis and liver cancer, diabetes, cardiomyopathy, and skin hyperpigmentation. If left untreated and allowed to progress, this disease can be fatal. Homozygotes for the allele can develop overt disease; heterozygotes do not, but may accumulate more iron than normal. Secondary hemochromatosis is iron overload due to another disease, condition, or lifestyle factor, such as frequent blood transfusions to treat beta-thalassemia major and other hereditary or acquired anemias, chronic hemolysis, or excessive iron intake (this iron may be contained in foods or supplements).

Hodgkin's Lymphoma

Hodgkin's lymphoma (Hodgkin's disease) is a primary malignant tumor of the lymph nodes characterized by the presence of Reed-Sternberg (R-S) cells. These are large multinucleated cells (shown in the image) or cells with a bilobate nucleus resembling an owl's eyes. R-S cells are the hallmark of Hodgkin's lymphoma, which cannot be diagnosed if these cells are absent. R-S cells are also seen in reactive lymphadenopathies resulting from infectious mononucleosis (Epstein-Barr virus). Depending on the patient's sex and age and the stage and subtype of the disease (classical Hodgkin's lymphoma and nodular lymphocyte-predominant Hodgkin's lymphoma), it is variously treated with radiation and/or chemotherapy, or with hematopoietic stem cell transplantation. The overall five-year survival rate is over 83 percent. Nevertheless, the estimated numbers of new cases of Hodgkin's lymphoma and associated deaths for 2012 are 9,060 and 1,190, respectively.

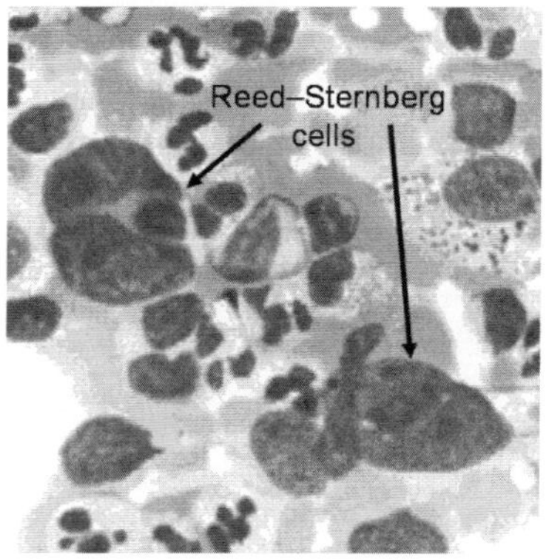

Von Willebrand Disease

Pseudohemophilia, or von Willebrand disease (vWD) as it is now called, is an inherited autosomal dominant coagulation disorder resulting from quantitatively insufficient or abnormal von Willebrand factor, which is an endothelial protein required for platelet aggregation. The disease usually presents as a relatively mild condition characterized by bruising, recurrent nosebleeds, heavy menstruation, and prolonged or excessive bleeding during childbirth, surgery, or dental work. However, in severe cases, vWD can be life-threatening. Type 1 vWD is the mildest and most common form of the disease. Type 2 usually appears during childhood; the symptoms are generally more severe than those seen with type 1. Type 3 is the most severe form of vWD, and can be life-threatening. A non-inherited acquired form of vWD can be precipitated by certain cancers, scleroderma, lupus, autoimmune disease, toxic environmental chemicals, and certain medications.

Osteoporosis

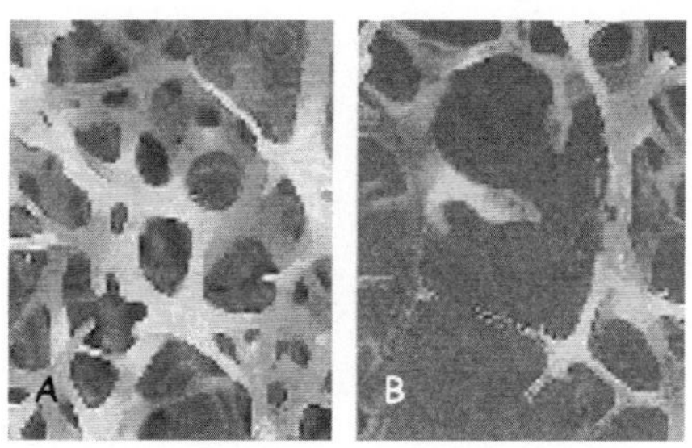

Atherosclerotic Lesions on Arteries

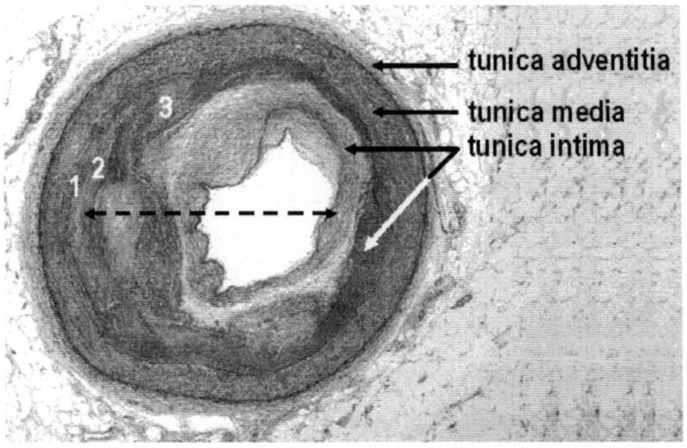

Microbiology

Human Blood

Blood is the only fluid tissue in the body. It consists of blood cells, platelets, and other formed elements that are capable of movement because they are suspended in a fluid plasma. Plasma consists of about 90 percent water, and the remaining 10 percent is comprised of nutrients, gases, electrolytes and buffering ions, glucose, amino acids and various proteins (including immunoglobulins and lipoproteins), and the products of cellular metabolism. Blood is the transportation system for the body, conveying oxygen and nutrients to tissues and cells, CO_2 and metabolic wastes to the kidneys and lungs for elimination, and hormone messengers from endocrine cells to their target tissues and cells. The blood regulates body temperature by absorbing and redistributing heat, and it maintains body pH and proper fluid volume. Excessive blood loss from injury is prevented by clotting mechanisms, and the blood fights infection by means of humoral and cell-mediated immune responses.

Formed Elements of the Blood

The formed elements of the blood are the anucleate erythrocytes (red blood cells), leukocytes (white blood cells), and platelets, tiny cytoplasmic fragments from megakaryocytes that function in blood clotting. All elements are formed in the red bone marrow. Erythrocytes are biconcave disks containing huge amounts of hemoglobin, the iron-bearing protein that carries oxygen in the blood. Erythrocytes circulate in the blood for 120 days or so before they are destroyed in the spleen and their contents are recycled. Between two and three million erythrocytes are created and destroyed every second. Leukocytes include neutrophils, eosinophils, basophils, lymphocytes (the cells classified as B or T cells depending on whether they mature in the spleen or the thymus gland that are involved in humoral immunity), monocytes, and the large amoeboid macrophages derived from monocytes that engulf and digest various pathogens and cellular debris.

Innate and Adaptive Immune Responses

The generalized innate immune response is triggered when widely occurring antigens on invading microorganisms are identified by pattern recognition receptors, or when inflammatory cytokines are released by the tissues. Innate immune responses are nonspecific, and do not confer long-lasting immunity. In contrast, the antigen-specific adaptive immune response involves recognition of very specific non-self antigens. It also involves the mobilization of killer T cells or the production of antibodies by B lymphocytes that are specifically tailored to bind to recognized foreign antigens. The antibodies are maintained in perpetuity (or at least for a very long period) by memory cells, which are quickly mobilized in the event of a subsequent infection by the same pathogen.

Humoral Immunity

Humoral immunity is part of the adaptive immune response. It is mediated by antibodies released by B lymphocytes, which are derived from the hematopoietic stem cells in the bone marrow (where they mature). When an antigen-bearing foreign body invades the body, a macrophage of the reticuloendothelial system engulfs it. It then presents a fragment of the antigen along with its own (self) antigens on its surface bound up with a major histocompatibility complex type II. One or more helper T cells bind to the foreign antigen and release cytokines that stimulate both the humoral and cellular immune responses. In humoral immunity, these cytokines activate antigen-specific B cells. When co-stimulated by another antigen-presenting cell or by $CD4^+$ and/or T-helper 2 cells, these B cells transform into plasma cells that release antibodies. These antibodies then bind to their respective antigens on invading foreign bodies and flag them for destruction. Some of the activated

B cells become persistent memory cells that elicit an enhanced secondary immune response to subsequent infections by the same pathogen.

Cellular Immunity

Cell-mediated immunity involves T lymphocytes that are derived from hematopoietic stem cells in the bone marrow and mature in the thymus gland. Two-thirds to three-fourths of mature T lymphocytes circulate in the blood; the rest are located in the spleen and lymph nodes. In the presence of foreign pathogens, these T cells are activated by helper T cells (which are themselves stimulated by antigen-presenting macrophages). They proliferate rapidly to produce cytotoxic T cells, which release perforin molecules that attack invading foreign cells and kill them. Natural killer cells and macrophages are also activated and recruited into this process.

Major Pathways in Humoral and Cellular Immunity

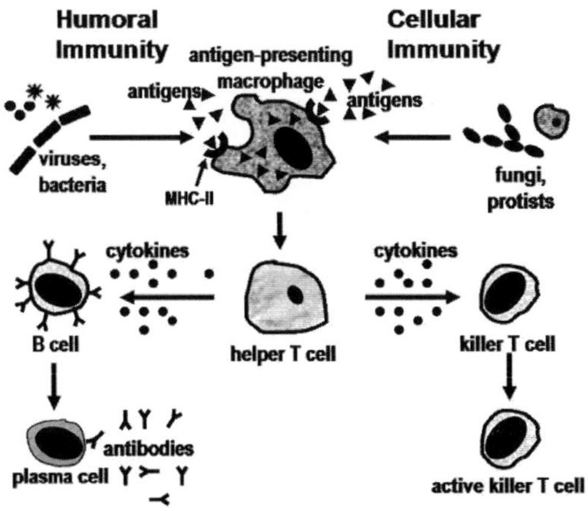

Antibodies

Antibodies or immunoglobulins are high molecular weight, Y-shaped glycoproteins produced by specialized B lymphocytes in the humoral immune system. They identify and attach to the complementary site of specific protein antigens on invading bacteria, viruses, or other xenobiotic (foreign) objects such as inhaled mold spore toxins. The B cells engulf the foreign object, break the antigen into fragments, and present it on the surface complexed with major histocompatibility class II (MHC-II) molecules. When co-stimulated by a dendritic cell subsequently presenting the same antigen, the B cell transforms into a plasma cell, which produces and releases many copies of the antigen into the blood or lymph. Certain T-helper cells can augment this co-stimulation. Each antibody combines with and neutralizes a specific antigen, and flags it for destruction by macrophages. Some of these B cells become memory cells. When re-exposed to the antigen, these cells produce a new round of soluble antibodies to attack and neutralize the invading pathogen or molecule.

Placental Mammalian Antibody Isotypes

The five antibody (immunoglobulin) isotypes of placental mammals are IgA, IgD, IgE, IgG, and IgM. IgAs are found in the mucosae of the gut, the respiratory tract, and the urogenital tract, as well as in saliva and tears. They protect against initial pathogen colonization. IgD is an unexposed B cell antigen receptor that activates basophils and mast cells. IgE protects against helminth infections and triggers the release of histamine from mast cells and basophils. It is involved in allergic reactions. IgGs are the primary mechanism underlying antibody-based immunity against pathogens. Maternal IgGs confer passive immunity to the fetus. IgM on the surface of B cells attacks pathogens before adequate amounts of IgGs have been produced.

Antigen-Antibody Complex

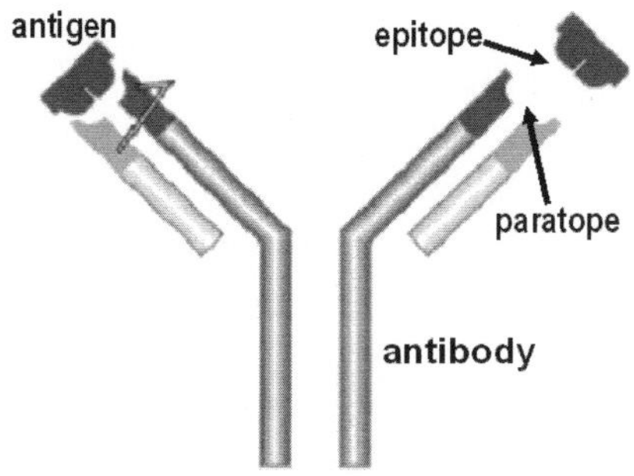

Complement System in the Immune Response

The complement system is part of the innate immune system involving 30 or so inactive circulating proteins (zymogens). When stimulated by certain triggers, these zymogens are cleaved by proteases into active proteases, which in turn cleave other proteins and release cytokines that initiate a cleavage cascade. This cascade eventually activates the membrane attack complex (MAC) to kill invading bacteria. The MAC creates transmembrane channels that lyse and destroy the invading cell. The complement system provides an initial defense while the antibody-mediated system is revving up. Then, the antibodies search out and target the invading pathogens, while the MAC attacks and kills them.

Biochemical Pathways

Three biochemical pathways are involved in the activation of the complement system. The classical pathway involves IgG or IgM antibodies complexed with the antigen. The alternative pathway is activated by IgA-antigen complexes, as well as by certain components of the bacterial cell wall, which can activate the complement system without antibodies being present. The lectin pathway is mediated by mannose-binding protein, a lectin that identifies and binds to mannose-containing carbohydrates found in bacterial cells but not in host cells.

Hypersensitivity Reactions

Hypersensitivity reactions are abnormal immune system responses to nonpathogenic foreign or host (self) antigens, which can cause uncomfortable or even fatal reactions (anaphylaxis). Allergies are abnormal and exaggerated responses to nonpathological antigens normally present in the environment. These abnormal reactions only occur when the individual has been previously exposed to the allergen(s). Autoimmune reactions involve a failure to recognize the body's own components as parts of the self. As a result, the immune system launches an attack against its own cells.

Allergic Reactions

Allergic responses to normal environmental allergens involve overstimulation of specific leukocytes known as mast cells and basophils by immunoglobulin e (IgE). Allergic reactions can lead to inflammatory responses ranging from mild but uncomfortable urticaria and eczema (contact and atopic dermatitis) and allergic rhinitis and conjunctivitis (hay fever), to more severe asthma attacks, or even life-threatening anaphylaxis. Allergic reactions require previous exposure to the allergen. Mild allergic responses like hay fever (which occurs due to exposure to pollen, mold, dust, and pet dander) and contact dermatitis (which occurs due to exposure to poison oak and poison ivy, *Toxicodendron* spp.) are common. More severe allergic reactions include asthma (which is characterized by inflammation of the airways) and bronchospasm (which involves airflow obstruction). Very severe and even life-threatening anaphylactic reactions can occur in individuals who are hypersensitive to certain foods, medications, or hymenopteran (bee and wasp) venoms.

Methods to Determine Sensitivity to Allergens

A RAST (radioallergosorbent test) for allergen-specific IgE antibodies is a blood test used to determine whether or not an individual is allergic to one or more allergens. A skin allergy test involves exposing the individual to tiny amounts of various allergens by scratching or pricking the skin to see what, if any, reactions (e.g., rash, itching, etc.) occur. Contraindications to a scratch, prick, or patch skin test include eczema that is severe enough to prevent such testing or the danger of major medical complications if an antihistamine medication is withheld. The RAST is performed *in vitro* on blood taken from the patient, and does not carry the potential hazards of an *in vivo* challenge. An elimination test is typically used to test for food allergies. Suspected food items are removed from the diet for a period of time and then reintroduced one at a time to see if allergic reactions occur.

Autoimmune Reactions

Autoimmune disorders arise when the immune system misidentifies the body's own cells and tissues as foreign and mounts an autoantibody attack against them. Autoimmune diseases and their targets include autoimmune hemolytic anemia (red blood cells), Graves' disease (thyroid), Hashimoto thyroiditis (thyroid), multiple sclerosis (myelin sheaths of neurons in the brain and spinal cord), rheumatoid arthritis (joints, lungs, nerves, skin, and heart), ulcerative colitis (colon and rectum), type 1 diabetes (pancreatic beta cells), and pernicious anemia, which results in impaired vitamin B_{12} uptake (gastric mucosa).

Efficacy of Vaccinations

Vaccination involves the administration of an antigen or antigenic mimic to stimulate an adaptive immunity to a particular disease. Vaccines can employ (1) intact pathogens that are non-infective (inactivated) or have lowered infectivity (attenuated); (2) purified antigenic components of a pathogen, such as viral proteins; or (3) toxoids, bacterial endotoxins that are modified to eliminate their toxicity while retaining their immunogenicity. The efficacies of various vaccines vary widely, and many are highly controversial because of disputed efficacies and serious adverse side effects. Despite disclaimers, serious adverse effects from vaccines are not rare. Because many vaccines are only partially effective, adjuvants—typically aluminum, squalene, or thimerosal (50 percent ethyl mercury)—are added to augment the immune response. Some vaccines confer lifelong immunity; others are only marginally effective or must be periodically readministered. Individual immune systems vary widely in terms of their responses to a vaccine challenge, and not everyone achieves the same level of immunity. Some persons remain nonresponders even after repeated vaccinations.

Prokaryotes and Eukaryotes

Prokaryotic cells have a plasma membrane with a protein-to-phospholipid ratio that is greater than three to one. In eukaryotes, this ratio is very close to one to one. Prokaryotes have no nucleus or other membrane-bound organelles, and their 70S ribosomes are smaller than the 80S ribosomes of eukaryotes. N-formylmethionine is the initiating amino acid of prokaryotic transcripts; eukaryotes employ methionine. The circular DNA strand of prokaryotes is loosely contained in the cytoplasm. Eukaryotic DNA is complexed with histones and packaged inside chromosomes. Prokaryotic cells reproduce through budding or binary fission; eukaryotic cells exhibit cellular division involving mitosis (somatic cells) or meiosis (germ cells) and cytokinesis. Bacterial and archaeal flagella consist of helical filaments that rotate like propellers powered by a rotary engine driven by the flow of protons down a concentration gradient. Archaeal and eukaryotic flagella are powered by ATP hydrolysis. The process involved in this hydrolysis is unknown.

Spirochaete

Spirochaetes are long, helically coiled, gram-negative, chemoheterotrophic bacteria with distinctive axial filaments (flagella). These filaments run the length of the organism within the periplasmic space, and are enclosed in an outer sheath. Spirochaetes include both aerobic and anaerobic as well as free-living and parasitic forms. Some are virulently pathogenic [e.g., *Treponema pallidum* subsp. *pallidum* (syphilis) and *Borrelia burgdorferi* (*sensu stricto*), which causes Lyme disease].

Bacterial Cell

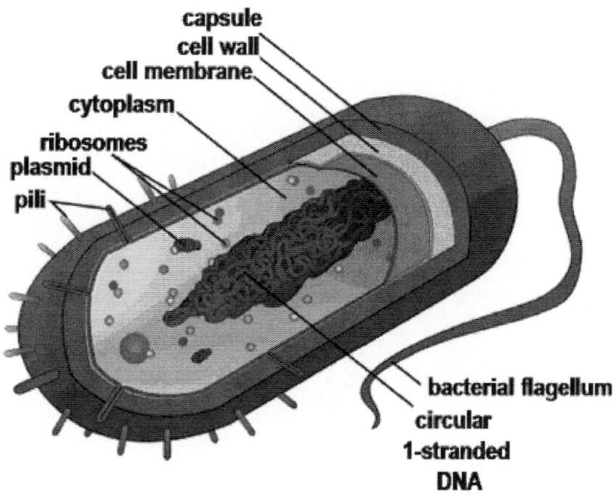

Staphylococci

The genus *Staphylococcus* includes a number of species of spherical, gram-positive, facultatively anaerobic (can function either aerobically or anaerobically) bacteria that form grapelike clusters and produce catalase (an enzyme that promotes clot formation). A dangerous human pathogen is methicillin-resistant *S. aureus* (MRSA), which has become resistant to the anti-staph antibiotics. Most MRSA infections occur in hospital patients and staff, nursing home residents, and dialysis patients, but community-acquired MRSA is becoming an increasing problem. Food poisoning, which can be life-threatening, is commonly due to infection by strains of *Staphylococcus*.

Pathogenic Bacteria

Most bacteria can be beneficial, but many cause serious diseases. In addition to spirochaetes and staphylococci, important pathogens include species and strains in the following genera: *Mycobacterium*, *Streptococcus*, *Pseudomonas*, *Yersinia* (e.g., *Y. pestis*, which causes plague), *Clostridium* (*C. tetani* and *C. botulinum*, which cause tetanus and botulism poisoning, respectively), *Legionella* (*L. pneumophila*, which causes Legionnaires' disease), and many others. *Escherichia coli*, a normal component of the gut microflora, has some virulently pathogenic strains, which cause serious and even fatal infections. Upper respiratory infections, exacerbations of COPD, and cases of acute otitis media (AOM) are commonly caused by *Hemophilus influenzae* (commonly called "H. flu" in medical circles), *Streptococcus pneumoniae*, and *Moraxella catarrhalis*. Half of the world's population is infected with *Helicobacter pylori*, the causative agent of peptic and duodenal ulcers and gastritis. This pathogen is also associated with an increased risk of gastric and duodenal cancers. However, 80 percent of infected individuals remain asymptomatic.

Classifications of Bacteria

Bacteria can be grouped according to shape. Bacilli are rod-shaped bacteria (*Escherichia* and *Salmonella*), cocci are spherical bacteria (*Streptococcus* and *Staphylococcus*), spirochaetes are spiral bacteria with flexible cell walls and axial filaments (*Treponema* and *Borrelia*), and spirilla are spiral bacteria with rigid cell walls and polar flagella (*Spirillum* and *Campylobacter*). Bacteria can also be classified according to their staining properties. Gram-positive bacteria stain blue or violet with crystal violet dye, while gram-negative bacteria appear red or pink with crystal violet dye. Bacteria may be classified as facultative or obligate aerobes or anaerobes, and may also be classified as autotrophic or heterotrophic.

Cell Wall of Gram-Positive Bacteria

The cell wall of gram-positive bacteria consists of many polymer layers of peptidoglycan connected by amino acid bridges. The peptidoglycan polymer is composed of an alternating sequence of N-acetylglucosamine and N-acetylmuramic acid. Peptidoglycan constitutes 90 percent of the cell wall of gram-positive bacteria.

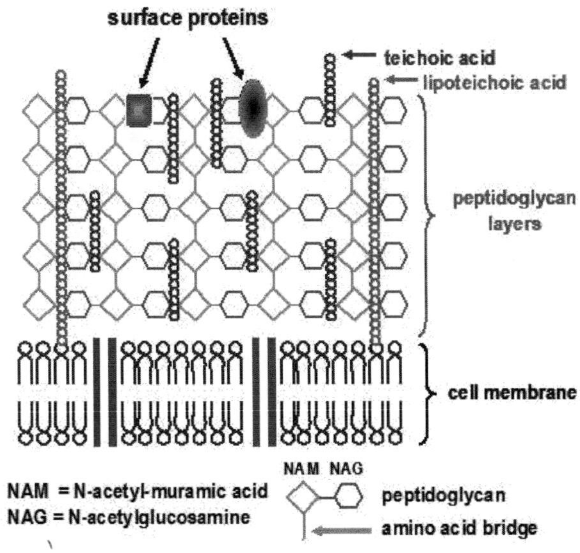

Cell Wall of Gram-Negative Bacteria

The cell wall of gram-negative bacteria is much thinner. Peptidoglycan comprises only 20 percent of the cell wall. Gram-negative bacteria have two unique regions surrounding the outer plasma membrane: the periplasmic space and the lipopolysaccharide layer (LPS). The periplasmic space separates the outer plasma membrane from the peptidoglycan layer. It contains proteins, which destroy potentially dangerous foreign matter that gets into this space. The lipopolysaccharide layer is located adjacent to the exterior peptidoglycan layer. It is a phospholipid bilayer with a construction similar to that of the cell membrane, and it is attached to the peptidoglycan by lipoproteins. The lipid portion of the LPS contains a toxic substance called lipid A, which is responsible for most of the pathogenic affects associated with harmful gram-negative bacteria. Polysaccharides that extend out from the bilayer also contribute to the toxicity of the LPS. The LPS, the lipoproteins, and the associated polysaccharides together form what is known as the outer membrane.

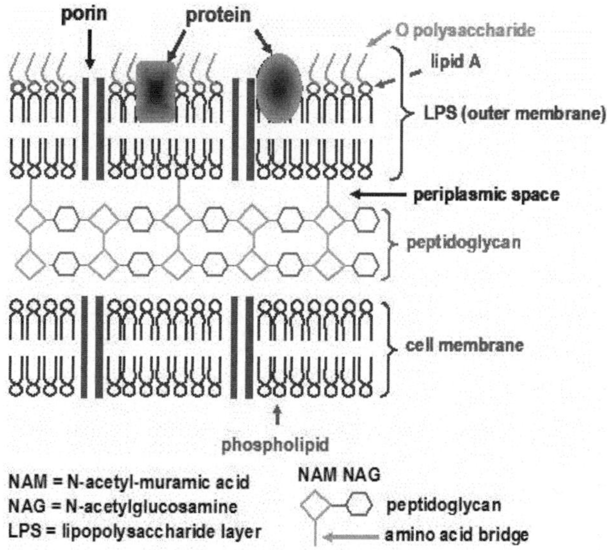

β-Lactam Antibiotics

β-lactam antibiotics include the penicillins and their derivatives, cephalosporins, monobactams, and carbapenems. They inhibit the synthesis of the peptidoglycan layer of bacterial cell walls in both gram-positive and gram-negative bacteria. Many of these pathogens have developed β-lactamases that attack the antibiotic's β-lactam ring. This can often be overcome by combining the antibiotic with clavulanic acid or another β-lactamase inhibitor.

Macrolide Antibiotics

Macrolides (e.g., erythromycin, clarithromycin, and azithromycin) are antibiotics whose action is based on a macrolide ring, which binds to the 50S bacterial ribosomal subunit and blocks the action of peptidyltransferase. This prevents the formation of the peptide bond between the peptidyl attached to the tRNA and the next amino acid. Ketolides and fluoroketolides (e.g., telithromycin, clarithromycin, and solithromycin) are related to macrolides. Both have two ribosomal binding sites. They are used to treat macrolide-resistant bacteria. Macrolides suppress the activity of CYP3A4 microsomal enzymes and, because they undergo enterohepatic recycling, can lead to toxic accumulations in the body.

Fluoroquinolones

Quinolones are broad-spectrum antibiotics that act by binding to and inhibiting bacterial DNA gyrase (a type II topoisomerase) and/or topoisomerase IV. This in turn inhibits DNA replication and transcription. Most of the quinolones used in clinical practice are fluoroquinolones (e.g., ciprofloxacin, gemifloxacin, levofloxacin, and gatifloxacin), which have a fluorine atom attached to the central ring system. Quinolones readily enter cells and therefore are often used to treat intracellular pathogens such as *Legionella pneumophila* and *Bacillus anthracis.* Fluoroquinolones preferentially target DNA gyrase over topoisomerase IV in *Escherichia coli.* These targets are reversed in *Staphylococcus aureus* and *Streptococcus pneumoniae.*

Tetracycline

Tetracycline and its derivatives (e.g., doxycycline and minocycline) are four-ring antibiotics that bind to the 30S subunit of bacterial ribosomes that interfere with protein synthesis. They block the attachment of charge aminoacyl-tRNA to the ribosomal A site and prevent amino acids from attaching to the growing peptide chain. They are used to treat infections of the respiratory tract, urinary tract, sinuses, and middle ear. They are also used to treat *Chlamydia* and *Helicobacter pylori* infections and anthrax exposure that is due to inhalation of the pathogen. Finally, tetracycline and its derivatives can be given to patients who are allergic to β-lactams and macrolides.

Bacterial Resistance to Antibiotics

Bacterial resistance to antibiotics can involve (1) inactivation of the antibiotic, (2) alterations in the target site that make the drug less effective, and (3) decreased access to the target site. β-lactamases cleave the lactam ring of β-lactam antibiotics. To inactivate the drug, gram-positive bacteria release large amounts of β-lactamases into their surroundings. Gram-negative bacteria use much smaller amounts of β-lactamases that are confined to the periplasmic space. Acetylation, phosphorylation, or adenylation by resistance enzymes in gram-positive and gram-negative bacteria inactivate aminoglycosides. Alterations to the target site include changes in DNA gyrase that confer resistance to quinolones and alterations to ribosomal RNA, which leads to resistance to macrolides and clindamycin. Vancomycin resistance involves alterations in a cell wall peptide. Gram-negative bacteria can block access to the target site through modifications to porin channels in their outer membrane that prevent access by all classes of antibiotics. Resistance to macrolides, tetracyclines, and quinolones commonly involves enhanced efflux mechanisms that expel the drug from the bacterial cell.

Genetic Resistance to Antibiotics

Genetic resistance to antibiotics can be intrinsic, involving mutations in innate DNA (vertical transfer). In most instances, though, bacteria develop such resistance by obtaining new genetic material from outside sources (horizontal transfer). Resistance mutations occur in one out of every 10^8–10^9 bacteria during an infection. The extreme growth rate of bacteria means that resistance develops quickly in a bacterial population. Resistance genes are horizontally acquired by importing foreign chromosomes, plasmids, or transposons. Plasmids transfer resistance genes within a bacterial class. Transposons exchange resistance genes between a wide range of bacterial species and strains. This can involve the direct transfer of genes by conjugation (plasmids and transposons), transformation (the uptake of free DNA from the surroundings), or the introduction of outside genetic material by bacteriophages (transduction). Resistance to sulfonamides and trimethoprim may involve overproduction of the target site to overwhelm the antibiotic's effect.

Conjugation, Transformation, and Transduction

Conjugation involves the transfer of plasmids—extrachromosomal DNA fragments—from a donor to a recipient bacterium. This occurs only between strains of the same or closely related species. Transformation is gene transfer resulting from the uptake of naked DNA from a donor cell by a recipient cell. *Bacillus*, *Haemophilus*, *Neisseria*, and *Pneumococcus* species, for example, can acquire DNA from the environment and incorporate it into their own genomes. Transduction involves the transfer of DNA from one infected bacterium to another by a bacteriophage. DNA fragments from an infected bacterial cell may become incorporated into the replicating virus and subsequently transferred to a new bacterial host. Here, the DNA fragments may undergo recombination with the host genome, giving the host cell new properties.

Bacterial Pathogenicity

Bacteria cause disease by two major mechanisms. The first is invasiveness, which refers to the ability of bacteria to invade the cells and tissues of their host. Invasiveness involves initial colonization and multiplication, the release of extracellular invasions that facilitate penetration into the host cell, and bypass mechanisms to overcome the host's defenses. The second mechanism is toxicogenesis, which refers to the production of toxins. Toxicogenesis can involve the release of exotoxins or endotoxins. Exotoxins released by pathogenic bacteria may act at distant sites from the focus of infection. Endotoxins are associated with the lipopolysaccharide portion of the outer membrane in gram-negative bacteria. However, endotoxins are typically liberated by the host's defenses or by antibiotics that lyse the invading bacteria, and may therefore also act at distant sites.

Infectious Dose and Lethal Dose

The 50 percent infectious dose, or ID_{50}, is the number of invading pathogens required to establish an infection in one-half of the hosts that are exposed to the pathogens. For some pathogen-host combinations, the ID_{50} may be quite high, while for others very few bacteria are needed to establish infection and/or disease. The 50 percent lethal dose, or LD_{50}, is the number of invading pathogens required to kill half of the host organisms exposed to the pathogens.

Bacterial Resistance to Host Defenses

Invading bacteria elicit immediate and nonspecific inflammatory and phagocytic responses by the host. This is followed by secondary, highly specific, antibody-mediated immune (AMI) and cell-mediated immune (CMI) responses involving the presentation of bacterial antigens by antigen-presenting cells. AMI and CMI responses are the host's main defenses against extracellular and intracellular pathogens, respectively. Both AMI and CMI responses occur once epithelial surfaces have been breached by bacteria. To ward off these defenses, bacteria employ a number of mechanisms, including increased tolerance to antigens due to persistent high levels of antigen, molecular mimicry, antigenic disguise (e.g., coagulase and protein A of *Staphylococcus aureus* and the fibronectin coat of *Treponema pallidum*), persistence of the pathogen at sites that are inaccessible to host defenses, and antigenic variability.

Transmission of Pathogenic Organisms

The transmission of pathogenic organisms and viruses can occur through physical contact with contaminated surfaces, ingestion of contaminated foods or fluids, contact with infected body fluids, and inhalation. Pathogenic organisms may also be transmitted via vectors, such as arthropods and other organisms. Due to their inherent virulence, primary pathogens cause infection and disease in healthy hosts. Opportunistic pathogens may be normally benign, but may produce disease in individuals whose resistance is diminished for any number of reasons. Pandemics are disease outbreaks affecting a great many people over wide geographic areas (continent-wide or global). Newly emergent diseases have resulted from human encroachment into previously pristine habitats that contain new pathogens and their vectors, urbanization and uncontrolled crowding of people in locations with unsanitary conditions, contaminated food and water supplies, and rapid international transportation of people and pathogens on modern carriers (ships and aircraft).

Food-Borne Bacterial Diseases

The most common food-borne bacterial pathogens are *Campylobacter jejuni*, *Clostridium perfringens*, *Salmonella* spp., and enterohemorrhagic and other strains of *Escherichia coli*. *Vibrio cholerae* infections can become epidemic when natural disasters such as floods and hurricanes affect estuaries. In such circumstances, cholera is commonly contracted from drinking water that contains naturally occurring *V. cholerae* or is contaminated by infected feces. Brucellosis from

Brucella melitensis is acquired through contact with infected body fluids from infected cattle and other livestock. It was a major problem in the past when people regularly consumed raw milk and milk products made from it, but has largely disappeared since pasteurization became the norm. Additionally, modern hygiene standards practiced by raw milk producers in areas where producing raw milk is still legal have reduced the incidence of brucellosis to almost zero.

Community-Acquired and Hospital-Acquired Bacterial Infections

Community-acquired infections are transmitted in the community at large, while nosocomial infections are acquired in hospital settings. Because bacterial resistance to antibiotics is widespread in hospitals, they have historically been the sites of exposure to resistant pathogens like hospital-acquired MRSA (HA-MRSA). However, because of the recent spread of resistant microbes in the community at large resulting from poor physician prescribing practices, patient noncompliance in taking complete doses of prescribed antibiotics, and other factors, community-acquired MRSA (CA-MRSA) is rapidly becoming a serious problem. HA-MRSA is typically multidrug resistant, and may only be susceptible to glycopeptides like vancomycin. CA-MRSA is often resistant to just one class of antibiotics, and is thus (for the time being at least) generally easier to treat than HA-MRSA.

Rickettsiae

Rickettsiae are tiny, gram-negative, highly pathogenic bacilli or cocci of the genera *Rickettsia* (spotted fever and typhus), *Orienta* (scrub typhus), *Coxiella* (Q fever), and *Bartonella* (trench fever and cat scratch disease). Except for *Bartonella*, which is facultative, all are obligate intracellular parasites of eukaryotic cells. They are transmitted through the bites of infected acarines (ticks and mites) or the feces deposited by infected lice, fleas, and sandflies in their bites or other skin abrasions. Many untreated human rickettsial infections have a high mortality.

Disease Reservoirs

The reservoir of a disease is the inanimate location (e.g., soil) or living host where the infectious agent survives long-term. Sciurids (squirrels and their kin) and Old World rats harbor *Yersinia pestis* (bubonic plague), which is transmitted by their ectoparasitic fleas. Opossums, armadillos, woodrats (*Neotoma* spp.), and other mammals harbor *Trypanosoma cruzi* (the protozoan parasite for Chagas disease). Chimpanzees, mangabeys, and nine-banded armadillos serve as reservoirs for leprosy. Both domestic and wild Carnivora species (skunks, foxes, dogs, wolves, coyotes, and raccoons) and Microchiroptera species (insectivorous bats) are the natural reservoirs for rabies and Australian bat lyssavirus. Megachiroptera species (fruit bats) are reservoirs for Ebola virus. Many opportunistic pathogens reside in healthy individuals without causing any symptoms, and only appear as diseases when the host becomes weakened or debilitated.

Transmission of Bacterial and Viral Diseases

Bacterial and viral infections are transmitted in a wide variety of ways: airborne respiratory and salivary secretions (pertussis, tuberculosis, bacterial and viral pneumonia, and common colds), skin contact with infected surfaces or body fluids (human papilloma virus and adenoviruses), sexual activity (syphilis, gonorrhea, chlamydia, HIV, hepatitis B and C, herpes simplex, and adenoviruses), fecal-oral transmission (cholera, typhoid fever, salmonellosis, adenoviruses, and poliomyelitis), penetration through wounds in the skin [tetanus, gas gangrene (*Clostridium* spp.)], animal vectors (typhus, Rocky Mountain spotted fever, Lyme disease, yellow fever, equine encephalomyelitis, dengue virus, and other related hemorrhagic fever viruses), and animal bites (rabies).

Viruses

Viruses are tiny (30–230 nm) infectious agents that can only replicate inside living cells. They are not living organisms, but nonliving particles called virions. They consist of a genome (either DNA or RNA) enclosed in a protein or glycoprotein capsid, which is coded for by the viral genome. They are sometimes also surrounded by a lipid envelope derived from the host cell plasmalemma. Possessing no machinery to transcribe and translate their genomes, they require the enzymes and organelles of a prokaryotic or eukaryotic cell in order to reproduce their own genomes and capsids. Viruses do undergo mutation and evolve through natural selection, but do not have a cellular grade of organization, the cell being the basic unit of life. Many viruses are highly pathogenic, and cause serious debilitation or death when they infect a host. Others have co-evolved with their hosts and are more or less benign.

Review Video: Viruses and Antiviral Drugs
Visit mometrix.com/academy and enter code: 984455

Infection of Cells by Viruses

Infecting viruses attach to specific receptors on the surface of the host cell, and are taken into the cell by endocytosis or through fusion with the plasma membrane (animal cells). Plants and fungi are infected through injury to the cell wall, and bacteriophages inject their genetic material directly into their bacterial host. Inside the host cell, the capsid separates from the viral genome and is transcribed and translated by the host cell's machinery. New virions subsequently spontaneously self-assemble and escape by lysing and killing the cell. Some viral genomes are incorporated into the host cell genome, where they may remain dormant as a provirus for a period and replicate whenever the host cell divides. At some point, they can form active virions and lyse the cell or escape by budding off from the host cell.

Virus Types

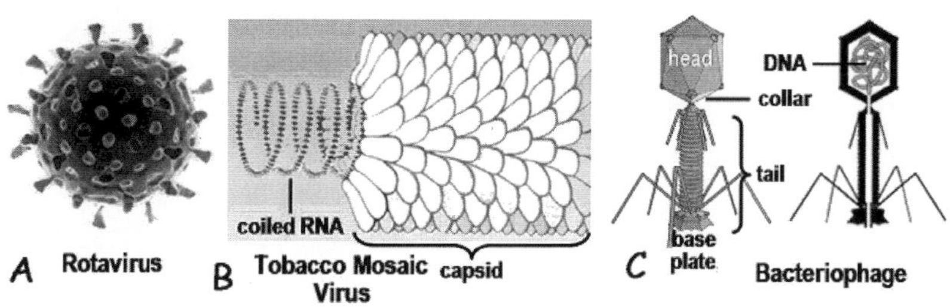

RNA Viruses

RNA viruses have genomes composed of single-stranded RNA (ssRNA) or double-stranded RNA (dsRNA). The vast majority of viruses are RNA viruses. A given viral genome can code for as few as two or more than a thousand different proteins. The host cellular machinery may synthesize some RNA virus proteins directly, without the need for transcription. However, retroviruses like HIV contain their own reverse transcriptase—an RNA-dependent DNA polymerase enzyme—to transcribe their RNA into a DNA intermediate. The transcribed DNA is then inserted directly into the DNA of the host genome, where it codes for viral proteins. The term ribovirus refers to all RNA viruses with the exception of retroviruses. Since viral RNA polymerases lack the proofreading capacity of DNA polymerases, RNA viruses exhibit exceptionally high rates of mutations.

Diseases Caused by Viruses

RNA viruses cause the vast majority of serious human diseases: hepatitis C, yellow fever, and West Nile virus (Flaviviridae); HIV (Retroviridae); SARS (Coronaviridae); influenza (Orthomyxoviridae);

measles, mumps, and Nipah viral encephalitis (Paramyxoviridae); poliomyelitis (Picornaviridae); rabies, European and Australian bat lyssaviruses, and vesicular stomatitis virus (Rhabdoviridae); Ebola and Marburg virus (Filoviridae); and hantavirus diseases, including hemorrhagic fever with renal syndrome (HFRS) and hantavirus pulmonary syndrome (HPS) (Bunyaviridae). Diseases caused by DNA viruses include smallpox (Poxviridae); hepatitis B (Hepadnaviridae); human papillomavirus (Papillomaviridae); and herpes simplex, human cytomegalovirus, and Epstein-Barr virus (Herpesviridae).

Double-Stranded RNA (dsRNA) and Single-Stranded (ssRNA) Viruses

RNA viruses employ RNA replicase to replicate themselves in a host cell. In dsRNA viruses, each strand is replicated to produce duplicate viral genomes and viral capsid proteins. The ssRNA viruses can be either positive or negative. The RNA in positive ssRNA viruses is the sense strand, which serves as the template for mRNA formed by RNA replicase. This mRNA then becomes a template for replication of the viral genome and viral proteins. The genome in negative ssRNA viruses is a nonsense strand, from which RNA replicase produces new viral genomes (nonsense RNA) and proteins. The single-stranded RNA of retroviruses is converted into double-stranded DNA by reverse transcriptase. This DNA is incorporated into the host cell genome, and is subsequently replicated during the cell cycle.

Viral Pathogenicity

The virulence of viruses is dependent upon their ability to: (1) enter a host cell and replicate inside that cell; (2) overcome host defenses; (3) cause temporary or permanent damage to the host through cell lysis, toxin production, and tumorigenic transformation of host cells; and (4) induce other cytoplasmic or nuclear alterations in host cells.

Antiviral Defenses Employed by Animal Hosts

Animal host defenses include nonspecific (innate) humoral and cellular mechanisms. Humoral mechanisms involve physical and chemical virucidal mechanisms that destroy virions. These humoral mechanisms include low pH produced by inflammation, enzymes, and mucus. Cellular mechanisms include nucleases, proteases, and interferon. Specific (acquired) host mechanisms include antibodies and activated phagocytes.

Fungal Diseases

Candida species are responsible for most yeast infections (candidiasis). They cause diseases ranging from mild oral thrush and vaginitis to potentially life-threatening systemic diseases, such as hepatosplenic candidiasis, *Candida* peritonitis, and systemic candidiasis (which has a mortality rate of between 30 and 40 percent). *Candida albicans* is part of the normal flora, but can become an invasive pathogen in immunocompromised persons or those taking antibiotics or immunosuppressive medications. *Aspergillus* spores are inhaled every day by most of us, but in immunocompromised or allergic individuals, they can cause allergic or invasive aspergillosis. Coccidiosis due to *Coccidioides immitis* or *C. posadasii* is common in the American Southwest, as well as in portions of Mexico, Central America, and South America. Athlete's foot is caused by the genus *Trichophyton*, as are onychomycosis (fungal infections of the nails). Other genera are also involved in nail disease. Histoplasmosis primarily affecting the lungs is caused by *Histoplasma capsulatum*.

Aflatoxin Produced by *Aspergillus*

Human beings inhale *Aspergillus* spores every day without any ill effects. However, *Aspergillus* can cause mild to life-threatening disease by producing mycotoxins, allergic responses, and local or systemic infections in persons with compromised immune status. *Aspergillus flavus* and *A.*

parasiticus produce aflatoxin—a potent toxin and carcinogen—and commonly contaminate grains and nuts, especially under environmental stresses such as excessive humidity or drought. It is found in the dairy products of animals fed contaminated grain. Toxic or chronic exposure can cause hepatic necrosis, which can lead to cirrhosis and hepatic carcinoma involving epigenetic methylation and suppression of the *p53* tumor suppressor gene.

Histoplasmosis

Histoplasmosis, caused by *Histoplasma capsulatum*, exists as an asymptomatic infection in most people, but infants and immunocompromised persons can develop a dangerous disease. *Histoplasma capsulatum* exists as mycelium at ambient temperatures, but develops as a yeast at body temperatures in mammals, where it causes histoplasmosis. It is endemic in the Ohio, Missouri, and Mississippi River valleys in North America, but is also widespread in Europe, parts of Africa, eastern Asia, and Australia. Birds are unaffected by the disease, but transmit the spores in their droppings. Active spores can remain in contaminated soil for years, making farmers and construction workers especially susceptible to infection.

Primary Pathogenic Fungi

Primary pathogenic fungi differ from opportunistic pathogenic fungi in the following ways: (1) they can actively invade tissues; (2) they exhibit thermal dimorphism (dimorphic growth patterns based on differences in temperature); (3) at ambient environmental temperatures, they exist in mycelial form; and (4) higher temperatures inside the bodies of their mammalian hosts cause them to grow as yeasts that produce enzymes, permitting their survival there. Truly pathogenic fungi cause disease regardless of the health status of the host, although sex, age, and race are important factors. These diseases are relatively rare, and are restricted to certain geographic areas.

Opportunistic Pathogenic Fungi

Opportunistic pathogenic fungi differ from primary pathogenic fungi in the following ways: (1) they have very low inherent virulence; (2) recovery from an infection confers no immunity to subsequent disease when resistance is diminished; (3) no thermal or other dimorphism is present; and (4) no differences in the expression of the disease exist due to sex, age, or race.

Sexual and Asexual Reproduction in Human Pathogenic Fungi

Opportunistic fungal infections have increased in recent decades due to HIV/AIDS host immunocompromisation, organ transplants, and cancer treatments. The three major human pathogenic fungi (*Candida albicans*, *Cryptococcus neoformans*, and *Aspergillus fumigatus*) all limit their access to sexual reproductive methods in order to maximize their fitness as pathogens inside their hosts. Yet, all retain their machinery for sexual reproduction, enabling them to sexually exchange genetic material in the face of stress imposed by new host species or antimicrobial therapy. Other pathogenic fungi also appear to retain their ability to reproduce sexually.

Main Host Defense Mechanisms Against Fungal Infections

A variety of host defense mechanisms provide protection against fungal infections. Nonspecific mechanisms include intact skin and mucus membrane barriers, as well as cell-mediated immune mechanisms involving fungicidal macrophages, neutrophils, and natural killer cells. These provide adequate defenses against opportunistic fungal infections of low virulence. Specific humoral and cell-mediated immune responses provide defenses against the more virulent pathogenic fungi. T lymphocytes sensitized to specific fungal antigens release activating lymphokines that mobilize macrophages, which are the major defense against systemic fungal infections.

Protozoal Parasites

Protozoa represent an artificial (non-natural) category of unicellular protists that belong to unrelated phyla. Major protozoal diseases include amoebiasis (amoebic dysentery), caused by *Entamoeba histolytica* in contaminated food and water; malaria, caused by several species of *Plasmodium* spread by *Anopheles* mosquitoes, the most virulent and dangerous being *P. falciparum*; giardiasis, caused by a diplomonad called *Giardia lamblia* in contaminated water; African sleeping sickness, caused by *Trypanosoma brucei* spread by tsetse fly bites; Chagas disease, caused by *T. cruzi* in the bites of reduviid bugs belonging to the genus *Triatoma*; trichomoniasis, a sexually transmitted protozoan, *Trichomonas vaginalis*, that causes vaginitis in women and burning micturition in men; and toxoplasmosis, due to *Toxoplasma gondii*, which usually produces no symptoms or causes a flu-like illness for a few weeks, after which it remains asymptomatic for life except in immunocompromised individuals.

Malaria

The recurrent, cyclic, and severe fevers, headaches, arthralgias, vomiting, and hemolytic anemia of malaria occur when multiplying *Plasmodium* merozoites lyse red blood cells and escape into the bloodstream to infect new erythrocytes. In severe cases of falciparum malaria, the disease can progress to splenomegaly, hepatomegaly, and renal failure due to hemoglobinuria ("blackwater fever"), leading to coma and death. Mortality rates of 20 percent are not uncommon with malaria infections, even with intensive treatment. Several drugs are used for both the prophylaxis and treatment of malaria: the quinine-based chloroquine (in cases where the parasite is still susceptible), mefloquine and amodiaquine, the tetracycline doxycycline, and an atovaquone-proguanil combination (Malarone®, GSK). Atovaquone selectively interferes with the parasite's electron transport chain, and proguanil inhibits its purine synthesis. IV artesunate in combination with a quinine-based drug is the treatment of choice for severe falciparum malaria.

Defenses

The first line of defense against malaria involves genetically inherited abnormal hemoglobin (sickle cell trait) and glucose-6-phosphatase deficiency (G6PD, or glycogen storage disease). G6PD exists in some 400 million people worldwide. Those with G6PD can suffer hemolytic anemia under oxidative stress, but the trait confers protection against falciparum malaria. Similarly, homozygotes for sickle cell disease (sickle cell anemia, sickle cell-hemoglobin C disease, and the sickle cell-beta-thalassemias) experience a lifelong struggle with pain, infections, anemia, and stroke, and are at a high risk of early death from complications. However, the heterozygotes remain largely asymptomatic, and are protected against falciparum malaria.

Giardiasis

Giardiasis is a severe diarrhea caused by the ingestion of *Giardia lamblia* cysts in contaminated water or person-to-person or sexual contact. Widespread contamination of rivers, waterways, lakes, and ponds is due to livestock, and particularly to aquatic rodents such as muskrats and beavers. Attacks may include severe abdominal cramps, vomiting, watery diarrhea (often alternating with constipation), and fever lasting several days. Treatment is 250 mg of metronidazole (Flagyl) taken three times a day for five days. Because of the disulfiram-like effects of metronidazole in irreversibly blocking aldehyde dehydrogenase, alcoholic beverages must be avoided during treatment and for several days afterwards to prevent a toxic buildup of acetaldehyde. Sanitation and hygiene practices are of little value in preventing giardiasis. Public water supplies in many cities in Colorado are contaminated with *Giardia* because of the beaver population, and residents cannot use the water for drinking, washing, or brushing their teeth.

Amoebiasis

Amoebiasis is usually caused by fecal-oral transmission of *Entamoeba histolytica*, but anal-oral transmission is also possible. The protozoan can also be transmitted by direct contact with contaminated objects. Infections can be asymptomatic (commensal) or produce mild diarrhea to full-blown dysentery with bloody and mucous stools. Fulminate amoebiasis can result in erosion of the gut wall (amoebic dysentery) or amoebic liver abscesses. It is endemic in many Third World regions where sanitation is minimal, or where human feces is used as a fertilizer. Complications can include perforations of the pericardium, pleural, and/or abdominal cavities; lung abscesses; and meningoencephalitis. It is usually treated with metronidazole, and the prognosis is generally good.

Helminth Parasites

Helminth parasites include flukes (class Trematoda) and tapeworms (class Cestoda), both of which belong to the phylum Platyhelminthes. They also include roundworms and microfilaria (phylum Nematoda). Trematode infections can be caused by blood flukes (*Schistosoma* spp.), liver flukes (*Clonorchis sinensis*), lung flukes (*Paragonimus westermani)*, and several different intestinal flukes, with the incidence of schistosomiasis being second only to malaria in Sub-Saharan Africa. Fully a quarter of the human population may be infected with the roundworm *Ascaris lumbricoides*, which causes ascariasis. These infections are particularly common in the tropics, where sanitation is poor. Trematode, cestode, and *Ascaris* infections are transmitted by the oral-fecal route. Microfilariae are transmitted by biting insect vectors. Lymphatic filariasis is caused by *Wuchereria bancrofti* (which can lead to elephantiasis) and *Brugia* spp. Subcutaneous filariases (onchocerciasis) is caused primarily by *Onchocerca volvulus* (river blindness).

Treatment

Helminth infections are treated with vermicides (which immediately kill the worms) and vermifuges (which incapacitate them, eventually resulting in their death). Only five drugs are available to treat all known helminth infections. Some, such as albendazole, are better than others for certain infections, like hookworm caused by the nematodes *Ancylostoma duodenale* and *Necator americanus*. Trichuriasis caused by the human tapeworm (*Trichuris trichiura*) affects one billion people worldwide. Infections are mainly seen in tropical Asia, Africa, and South America, but more than two million persons in the rural sections of the American Southeast are also infected. Mebendazole is highly effective against this parasite, but albendazole and iron are frequently added. Tapeworm (*Taenia solium*) infections are caused by the ingestion of eggs in contaminated water or the ingestion of encysted larvae in raw or undercooked meat or muscle tissue. Cestode infections are treated with praziquantel, albendazole, and/or nitazoxanide.

Human Ectoparasites

Common human ectoparasitic problems include scabies (intense itching from a burrowing mite, *Sarcoptes scabiei*), head lice (*Pediculus humanus capitis*, which transmit no disease and may confer resistance to body lice, which do), body lice (*Pediculus h. humanus*, which transmit several serious diseases: louse-borne typhus, louse-borne relapsing fever, trench fever, and possibly even bubonic plague), pubic lice (often intense itching from *Pthirius pubis*), and several serious diseases transmitted by ticks (Acari: Ixodidae). Tick-borne diseases are due to a variety of rickettsia and other bacteria, viruses, and protozoa, two or more of which can simultaneously be transmitted in a single tick bite. Diseases transmitted by ticks include Lyme disease and relapsing fever (*Borrelia* spp. transmitted by *Ixodes* spp. ticks), Rocky Mountain spotted fever (*Rickettsia rickettsii*: *Dermacentor* spp.), tularemia (*Francisella tularensis* transmitted by several genera of ticks and tabanid flies), and Colorado tick fever (a coltivirus transmitted by *Dermacentor andersoni*), among others.

Treatment Options for Human Ectoparasites

Treatments for scabies include lindane, permethrin, and more recently ivermectin, especially in infested community or institutional settings. Combining ivermectin, an anti-helminth agent that is also effective against arthropods, with topical agents is an approach used to combat crusted scabies. Lice are variously treated with topical OTC shampoos containing permethrin, and pyrethrins. If resistance has developed, the next options are prescription benzyl alcohol lotion, malathion, and lindane. Lindane can have serious neurological side effects, and lice are becoming increasingly resistant to it.

Genetic Factors Leading to Increased Drug Resistance in Malarial Parasites

Plasmodium falciparum, the organism responsible for the more virulent forms of malaria, has become increasingly drug-resistant. It first became resistant to chloroquine, and then to antifolate-based chemotherapy, which has led to increased use of mefloquine and artemisinin. However, in some areas, *P. falciparum* is resistant to all malaria treatments. Variations in human genes coding for cytochrome P-450 microsomal drug-metabolizing enzymes cause some ethnic populations to clear antimalarial agents more slowly than other groups. Parasites infecting hosts with slower clearance rates are exposed to sub-therapeutic levels of the drug for longer periods, which promotes selection for drug-resistant parasites.

Parasite's Defenses Against Host's Reaction to Trypanosomiasis Infection

Trypanosoma brucei (African sleeping sickness) survives by evading the host's immune responses. It does this by spontaneously changing the composition of variant-specific glycoproteins (VSGs) that completely cover the parasite. A given parasite will present approximately 10^7 identical VSGs to the host's antigenic-mediated response, while nearly a thousand different sets of identical antigens are simultaneously presented by many other individual trypanosomes. Thus, only a small fraction of the parasites are destroyed by the host's antibody response to one or several of the antigens presented.

Prions

Prions are infectious misfolded proteins. They are the only known infectious agents that lack genetic material (DNA or RNA). When they infect the brain and nervous tissues of their mammalian hosts, they induce the properly folded host proteins to assume the misfolded form of the prion. These induced misfolded proteins become new infectious prions in their own right. These misfolded proteins are extremely stable and resistant to denaturation, and thus accumulate in the host's nervous tissues. Here, they produce "spongy holes" and neuronal loss. Prion diseases, known as transmissible spongiform encephalopathies (TSEs), have long incubation periods. When the typical spongiform features and associated neuronal loss appear, however, progression is rapid and always fatal. TSEs include Creutzfeldt-Jakob disease in humans, bovine spongiform encephalopathy in cattle, scrapie in sheep and goats, and chronic wasting disease in North American deer. Prions have also been found in certain fungi, but do not appear to induce any disease state.

Reporting Communicable Diseases

In this country, the legislatures of the various states determine which communicable infectious diseases physicians, other health-involved authorities, and health agencies and institutions are required to report. Reporting cases of infectious diseases is critical for identifying and controlling outbreaks and preventing or ameliorating epidemics and pandemics. Such timely knowledge helps ensure the timely detection of and dissemination of information about food-borne and other disease outbreaks. It also allows for the mobilization of logistical resources for appropriate medical interventions and prevention (e.g., vaccine availability). Many of these diseases are also required to be reported to the US Centers for Disease Control and Prevention.

Communicable Diseases Reportable to the CDC

Nationally reportable diseases include AIDS, anthrax, West Nile virus, botulism, brucellosis, bubonic and pneumonic plague, chickenpox, coccidiomycosis, diphtheria, giardiasis, all sexually transmitted diseases, hepatitis A, B and C, leprosy, Lyme disease, malaria, measles, mumps, pertussis, poliomyelitis, human and animal rabies, rickettsial diseases (e.g., Rocky Mountain spotted fever), salmonellosis, SARS, tetanus, Q fever, tularemia, tuberculosis, VRSA, and others. These diseases are tabulated and summarized in the *MMWR Morbidity & Mortality Weekly Report published by the CDC.*

Epidemiological Terms

Some of the most common epidemiological terms include: (1) common source—when victims acquire an illness from the same source, such as a contaminated water supply; (2) endemic—a communicable or infectious disease that exists more or less continuously in a particular location or region; (3) outbreak or epidemic—an outbreak of an infectious disease that is greater or more widespread compared to what is normally seen in a given area or group of people over a particular time period; (4) disease cluster—an aggregation of cases in a given area or in a specific group of people over a specified time period, whether or not the number of cases is higher than normal; (5) pandemic—a disease outbreak that spreads to all areas of the world; (6) propagation—transmission of a communicable disease from person to person; and (7) zoonotic—an infectious disease endemic in an animal population (e.g., rabies and bubonic plague).

Routine Disease Surveillance

Health officials learn about most disease outbreaks through phone calls made by physicians, who are reporting several suspected cases of an illness to one another or to local health departments. Public health surveillance teams routinely collect, analyze, evaluate, and disseminate public health data reported by physicians, laboratories, and other health authorities to detect potential disease outbreaks early on. The CDC relies primarily on reports from local and state health agencies. Sentinel surveillance is carried out by designated institutions. It involves the collection and evaluation of data related to the epidemiology of specific diseases in certain geographic areas. CDC's FoodNet (Foodborne Diseases Active Surveillance Network) is a major component of its active surveillance of foodborne diseases that relies on work performed in more than 650 clinical laboratories. FoodNet conducts periodic surveys of these laboratories and physicians practicing within the designated area to evaluate their testing techniques, knowledge, and practices. CDC's national Waterborne Disease and Outbreak Surveillance System (WBDOSS) receives and evaluates data about waterborne disease outbreaks and single cases of these diseases.

Controlling Disease Outbreak

Controlling an outbreak of infectious disease involves the following steps: (1) ascertain the actual risk of an actual or potential outbreak; (2) define what constitutes a case, and identify new cases as they appear; (3) develop hypotheses about the inferred source(s) of the outbreak, and institute initial control measures; (4) test and reevaluate the hypotheses using surveillance data and/or special investigations; (5) adjust the hypotheses and control measures as needed; and (6) implement long-term control and prevention measures.

Emerging Infectious Diseases

An emerging infectious disease (EID) is a disease that appears in a population for the first time. The term may also refer to a disease that may have existed previously, but is now undergoing a rapid increase in incidence or an expansion of its range. Emerging infections now account for 12 percent of all human pathogens. A number of factors underlie the appearance of EIDs: (1) newly identified microorganisms or new strains of a previously known organism; (2) mutational changes in an existing organism resulting in new infections; (3) geographic spread of a known infection to new areas; (4) new infections resulting from changing ecological conditions favoring the spread of a pathogen; (5) re-emergent infections resulting from increasing drug resistance by the pathogen; and (6) the appearance of syndemics, which are aggregations of two or more synergistically interacting diseases in a population that exacerbate the effects of any or all of the diseases.

Environmental Changes Leading to EIDs

Lyme disease, hantavirus pulmonary syndrome (HPS), Lassa fever, and the filovirus hemorrhagic fevers (Marburg and Ebola viruses) emerged when humans encountered the arthropod vectors (Lyme disease) or the hosts of the causative pathogens more frequently than before or for the first time. Humans can be exposed to these arthropod vectors and hosts through coming into contact with rodents (HPS and Lassa fever), working with or eating infected monkeys, or coming into contact with the urine and feces of infected fruit bats (Marburg and Ebola viruses). The changing technologies of air conditioning and mass food production have led to the emergence of Legionnaires' disease and hemolytic uremic syndrome, respectively.

Emerging Hantaviruses

Hantaviruses are negative-sense RNA viruses in the family *Bunyaviridae*. Some of them cause rare but life-threatening hemorrhagic fevers with renal syndrome (HFRS) or hantavirus pulmonary syndromes (HPS), which have high mortality rates. Unlike most bunyaviruses, which are transmitted by insect vectors, hantaviruses are transmitted to humans through bites by wild rodents or through the inhalation of their aerosolized droppings or urine. Hantavirus hemorrhagic fever with renal syndrome outbreaks in Asia, northwestern Europe, Russia, and elsewhere have a 55 percent mortality rate. Sin Nombre virus is a newly encountered hantavirus in North America that causes life-threatening cardiopulmonary syndromes (HPS). It has a 60 percent mortality rate. Its host is the ubiquitous and common deer mouse, *Peromyscus maniculatus*, but other rodents can also carry this virus.

Mechanisms by Which Bacteria Develop Antibiotic Resistance

β-lactams—penicillin derivatives (penams), cephalosporins (cephems), cephamycins, and carbapenems—inhibit cell wall synthesis in a wide spectrum of gram-positive and gram-negative bacteria. Resistant bacteria overcome these agents by producing β-lactamases. These enzymes break the β-lactam's ring, thus deactivating its bacteriostatic mechanism. Bacterial penicillin-binding sites are altered in MRSA. Tetracyclines, macrolides, and ketolides (e.g., azithromycin, clarithromycin, and telithromycin) inhibit bacterial protein synthesis by reversibly binding to the P site on the 50S subunit of the bacterial ribosome. Bacterial macrolide resistance mainly involves post-transcriptional methylation of the 23S ribosomal RNA and/or enhanced activity of the ATP-driven efflux mechanisms that export the drug from the bacterial cell. Quinolones and their newer generation derivative fluoroquinolones (e.g., ciprofloxacin, levofloxacin, and norfloxacin) inhibit bacterial DNA gyrase (a topoisomerase II) that allows DNA coils to unwind and replicate. Alteration of the penicillin-binding site is seen in MRSA.

NBCE Practice Test

General Anatomy

1. Which of the following cavities are contained within the dorsal cavity?

a. Pelvic
b. Thoracic
c. Cranial
d. Abdominal

2. The deltoid tuberosity is found on the

a. radius.
b. humerus.
c. femur.
d. tibia.

3. Which of the following is considered a cartilaginous joint?

a. Distal tibiofibular joint
b. Elbow joint
c. Condyloid joint
d. Pubic symphysis

4. Which of the following muscles do NOT help to move the lower leg?

a. Sartorius
b. Flexor pollicis brevis
c. Vastus lateralis
d. Semitendinosus

5. Which of the following is an INCORRECT statement about the blood supply through the heart?

a. The left coronary artery is the dominant artery in the majority of the population.
b. The left ventricle is the chamber of the heart that works the hardest.
c. Veins deliver deoxygenated blood to the right atrium.
d. The sinoatrial node acts as the pacemaker for the heart.

6. The pancreas has both exocrine and endocrine functions. Which of the following is NOT secreted by the pancreas?

a. Insulin
b. Glucagon
c. Bile
d. Trypsin

7. The part of the lung where gas exchange occurs is the

a. alveoli.
b. bronchioles.
c. bronchi.
d. capillaries.

8. Where is the pituitary gland located?

a. Near the kidney
b. The ventral surface of the brain beneath the hypothalamus
c. In the front of the neck distal to the larynx
d. In the lower right quadrant near the large intestine

Spinal Anatomy

9. What are the bones called that protect the top of the cranium?

a. Occipital
b. Frontal
c. Parietal
d. Temporal

10. Which of the following muscles is NOT located in the back?

a. Latissimus dorsi
b. External abdominal oblique
c. Intertransversarii
d. Sternocleidomastoid

11. Which of the following is NOT a muscle of the rotator cuff?

a. Infraspinatus
b. Teres minor
c. Teres major
d. Subscapularis

12. Which of the following joints is considered to be a pivot joint?

a. Intervertebral
b. Atlantoaxial
c. Costovertebral
d. Atlanto-occipital

13. What is the lowest part of the brainstem called?

a. Medulla oblongata
b. Cerebrum
c. Pons
d. Cerebellum

14. Where is the least amount of cerebrospinal fluid (CSF) found?

a. Subdural space
b. Epidural space
c. Subarachnoid space
d. Spinal cord

15. Cranial nerve III is called

a. olfactory.
b. facial.
c. hypoglossal.
d. oculomotor.

16. Contraction and relaxation of the diaphragm muscle is regulated by a nerve located in the

a. brachial plexus.
b. cervical plexus.
c. lumbar plexus.
d. sacral plexus.

17. Which of the following is responsible for dynamic equilibrium?

a. Macula
b. Otoliths
c. Cupula
d. Crista ampullaris

Physiology

18. Which of the following is NOT a physiologic change expected during a sympathetic response?

a. Dilation of the cardiac vessels
b. Increase in glycogenolysis
c. Dilation of the blood vessels in the digestive tract
d. Increase in lipolysis

19. The type of muscle contraction used during the lifting of a weight in a bicep curl would be

a. concentric contraction.
b. eccentric contraction.
c. isotonic contraction.
d. isometric contraction.

20. What is a typical cardiac output?

a. 1000 mL/min
b. 2500 mL/min
c. 5000 mL/min
d. 7500 mL/min

21. Breathing that is temporarily halted after a normal expiration is called

a. dyspnea.
b. apnea.
c. hyperpnea.
d. eupnea.

22. Which of the following is NOT a step in the formation of urine?

a. Reabsorption
b. Filtration
c. Tubular secretion
d. Renal clearance

23. Which of the following is NOT a major function of the liver?

a. Metabolism of carbohydrates
b. Storage of bile
c. Breakdown of ammonia into urea
d. Filtering various toxins and waste products for removal from the body

24. Protein anabolism and fat mobilization are direct actions of which of the following hormones?

a. Prolactin
b. Oxytocin
c. Growth hormone
d. Adrenocorticotropic hormone

CHEMISTRY

25. The conversion of glucose to pyruvic acid is called

a. glycolysis.
b. glucogenesis.
c. gluconeogenesis.
d. glycogenolysis.

26. Where does gluconeogenesis mainly occur?

a. Mitochondria
b. Kidney
c. Myocyte
d. Liver

27. Which of the following fatty acids cannot be made in the body?

a. Arachidonic acid and erucic acid
b. Linoleic acid and alpha-linolenic acid
c. Oleic acid and eicosapentaenoic acid
d. Docosahexaenoic acid and palmitoleic acid

28. Where does protein digestion begin?

a. Ileum
b. Duodenum
c. Stomach
d. Jejunum

29. Which of the following hormones acts to counteract hypoglycemia?

a. Adrenaline
b. Epinephrine
c. Insulin
d. Glucagon

30. Bone pain and muscle weakness may be caused by a deficiency of

a. vitamin D.
b. vitamin C.
c. vitamin A.
d. niacin.

31. Which of the following is NOT a function associated with potassium?

a. Assisting with the electrical impulses in the heart
b. Antioxidant properties
c. Contractions of skeletal and smooth muscles
d. Contributing to pH balance in the body

32. Which of the following factors do NOT work to increase the basal metabolic rate?

a. Fever
b. Male gender
c. Higher amounts adipose tissue
d. Thyroid hormone

PATHOLOGY

33. Which of the following diseases is considered an autoimmune disease?

a. Duchenne muscular dystrophy
b. Type 1 diabetes
c. Alzheimer disease
d. Cancer

34. A biochemical inflammatory marker that may be indicative of cardiac disease risk is

a. high-sensitivity C-reactive protein.
b. angiotensin-converting enzyme.
c. erythrocyte sedimentation rate.
d. platelet count.

35. An example of an autosomal recessive genetic condition is

a. cystic fibrosis.
b. Huntington disease.
c. Parkinson disease.
d. Duchenne muscular dystrophy.

36. Which of the following is NOT an autoimmune disease?

a. Systemic lupus erythematosus
b. Multiple sclerosis
c. Rheumatoid arthritis
d. Polycystic kidney disease

37. Weight-bearing exercise, prevention of falls, and supplementation with calcium and vitamin D would be appropriate primary treatments for which disease?

a. Osteogenesis imperfecta
b. Osteoporosis
c. Osteomyelitis
d. Osteoarthritis

38. A stroke occurring on the right side of the brain may cause all of the following EXCEPT

a. left-sided weakness of the body.
b. memory loss.
c. vision impairment.
d. dysphagia.

39. Arthritis occurs as a result of damage to which of the following types of joints?

a. Synchondroses
b. Synovial
c. Synarthroses
d. Symphyses

40. Nephropathy, retinopathy, and neuropathy are potential microvascular complications of

a. diabetes mellitus.
b. diabetes insipidus.
c. coronary artery disease.
d. polycystic kidney disease.

41. A blood pressure reading of 142/98 is consistent with

a. normal blood pressure.
b. prehypertension.
c. stage 1 hypertension.
d. hypertensive crisis.

MICROBIOLOGY

42. Leukotrienes and interferons are examples of

a. antigens.
b. B cells.
c. cytokines.
d. phagocytes.

43. T cells and B cells are types of

a. phagocytes.
b. lymphocytes.
c. granulocytes.
d. antibodies.

44. Which of the following is an example of a bacterial disease transmitted by ticks?

a. Tuberculosis
b. E. Coli
c. Cholera
d. Rocky Mountain spotted fever

45. Which of the following is transmitted through the fecal-oral route?

a. Hepatitis A
b. Hepatitis B
c. Hepatitis C
d. All types of hepatitis

46. The most common form of waterborne illness in the United States is

a. E. Coli.
b. adenovirus.
c. giardiasis.
d. cryptosporidiosis.

47. What type of infection is caused by dermatophytes?

a. Fungal
b. Bacterial
c. Viral
d. Parasitic

48. Which of the flowing is NOT a characteristic of a group A streptococcal infection?

a. Strep throat
b. Impetigo
c. Pneumonia
d. No signs of illness

49. Which of the following agencies is responsible for assisting with the monitoring of public health, investigation into sources of disease outbreak, research, education, and strategies for prevention of disease and illness as well as being instrumental in emergency preparedness and response as it relates to natural disasters as well as acts of terrorism?

a. Food and Drug Administration
b. Centers for Disease Control and Prevention
c. Consumer Health and Safety Council
d. National Institutes of Health

50. Which of the following is an example of a reemerging disease?

a. Mumps
b. Chicken pox
c. Tetanus
d. Hepatitis A

Answer Key and Explanations

1. C: The human body contains two major cavities: the dorsal cavity and the ventral cavity. The dorsal cavity contains the cranial and spinal cavities. Dorsal refers to the back part of the body. The brain and spinal cord are within the dorsal cavity. The ventral cavity includes the mediastinum and diaphragm and the thoracic, pleural, abdominal, and pelvic cavities. Ventral refers to the front of the body. The main organs that are within the ventral cavity include the lungs, heart, trachea, thymus gland, liver, gallbladder, pancreas, intestines, spleen, kidneys, ureters, bladder, reproductive organs, and parts of the large intestines (sigmoid colon and rectum).

2. B: The upper extremity bones include the shoulder girdle, the upper and lower parts of the arms, the wrists, and the hands. The clavicle and the scapula make up the shoulder girdle. The upper arm bone is the humerus and the forearm includes the radius (on the thumb side) and the ulna (on the side of the little finger). The markings on the humerus include the head, anatomical neck, greater tubercle, lesser tubercle, intertubercular groove, surgical neck, deltoid tuberosity, radial groove, epicondyles, capitulum, trochlea, olecranon fossa, and coronoid fossa. The markings found on the radius include the head, radial tuberosity, and styloid process. The markings on the ulna include the olecranon process, coronoid process, trochlear notch, radial notch, head, and styloid process.

3. D: There are three main classifications of joints: synarthrosis, amphiarthrosis, and diarthrosis. Synarthrosis joints are fibrous joints that contain connective tissue to keep the joint close together. This type of joint can be subclassified into syndesmosis (ligaments that connect two bones), suture (found solely in the skull), and gomphosis (found in the mandible or maxilla and the roots of teeth). Synarthrosis joints are typically immovable or allow only very limited movement. Amphiarthrosis joints are considered cartilaginous joints that also allow limited movement but only in very select cases. An example of this is the pubic symphysis joint that expands slightly during the childbirth process. Diarthrosis joints are synovial joints that are freely movable. Synovial joints are further classified into uniaxial (hinge and pivot joints), biaxial (saddle, condyloid), and multiaxial (ball and socket, gliding joints). An example of a uniaxial joint is the elbow joint, a biaxial joint is the wrist joint, and a multiaxial joint is the shoulder or hip joint.

4. B: The muscles that help to move the lower leg are categorized within two main groups: the quadriceps femoris group and the hamstring group. The quadriceps femoris group includes the rectus femoris, vastus lateralis, vastus medialis, vastus intermedius, and sartorius. The femoral nerve regulates the muscle activity. The quadriceps group works to flex the thigh and extend the leg. The hamstring group consists of the biceps femoris, semitendinosus, and semimembranosus. The sciatic nerve regulates the muscle activity in the hamstring group. The hamstring group works to extend the thigh and flex the leg.

5. A: The heart contracts through the electrical conduction system. Impulses are released that cause the heart muscle to contract. There are four parts of the electrical conduction system: the sinoatrial (SA) node, which acts as the pacemaker, the atrioventricular (AV) node, the AV bundle, and the subendocardial branches. There are four chambers of the heart: the left and right atria and the left and right ventricles. Veins bring blood to the right atrium, then the blood travels to the right ventricle. From here the blood enters the pulmonary circulation in order to be oxygenated. The pulmonary vein brings the oxygenated blood to the left atrium. The oxygenated blood then enters the left ventricle to be pumped throughout the body through arteries. The left ventricle is the chamber of the heart that works the hardest. In approximately 50% of the population, the right coronary artery is the dominant artery. Narrowing of any of the coronary arteries leads to a reduction in oxygen, angina, and may lead to a heart attack.

6. C: The pancreas has two main functions: exocrine and endocrine. The endocrine function serves to help regulate blood glucose levels. Beta cells secrete insulin and alpha cells secrete glucagon. The exocrine function aids in the digestive process by secreting pancreatic enzymes from the acinar units of the pancreas. Proteases such as trypsin and chymotrypsin are secreted by the pancreas to aid in the digestion of protein. Lipase is secreted to help digest fat and amylase helps with the digestion of starches. Nucleases are also secreted for RNA and DNA digestion. Pancreatic secretions also include sodium bicarbonate for assistance with acid-base balance. Bile is secreted by the liver but is also necessary for the digestive process.

7. A: The trachea continues down from the larynx to the primary bronchi, which then enter the lungs. The right and left lungs are each divided into lobes. The left lung has two lobes (the superior and inferior) and the right lung has three lobes (superior, middle, inferior). The right and left bronchi continue to divide into secondary bronchi, then smaller bronchioles, and ultimately alveoli. This structure is referred to as the bronchial tree. It is within the grape-shaped alveoli that gas exchange of carbon dioxide for oxygen occurs. Surfactant is present within the alveoli to help retain shape and prevent collapse during the gas exchange. There are over 300 million alveoli within the lungs.

8. B: The pituitary gland is a very small endocrine gland measuring about 1.5 centimeters. It is located within the skull on the ventral surface of the brain just below the hypothalamus. The pituitary gland is divided into two parts: the anterior pituitary and the posterior pituitary. The anterior pituitary secretes growth hormone, adrenocorticotropic hormone (ACTH), thyroid-stimulating hormone, prolactin, luteinizing hormone, and follicle stimulating hormone. The posterior pituitary is considered to be an extension of the hypothalamus gland. This area serves to store and release antidiuretic hormone and oxytocin. Both of these hormones are produced in the hypothalamus, and nerve stimulation causes their release from the posterior pituitary.

9. C: The skeleton is divided into two parts: the axial and the appendicular skeletons. The parts of the body that are included in the axial skeleton include the head, neck, and torso. In the head, the parietal bones are the bones that protect the top of the cranium and are described as bulging. Other main bones around the skull include the frontal bone, temporal bones, occipital bone, sphenoid bone, and ethmoid bone. Facial bones including the upper and lower jaw, cheek, nose, hard palate, ear, orbits of the eye and the hyoid bone are part of the axial skeleton. In the torso area the vertebral column, sternum, and ribs are also part of the axial skeleton. There are 74 total bones in the axial skeleton as well as 6 very tiny bones within the middle ears. The appendicular skeleton consists of the bones of the arms and legs.

10. D: The sternocleidomastoid muscle is located in the neck and assists with chewing and facial expressions. There are a great number of muscles in the area of the back. There are superficial back muscles that help to move the head and limbs. Types of superficial muscles include the trapezius, deltoid, latissimus dorsi, and external abdominal oblique muscles. There are also deep back muscles that help to move the vertebral column and keep the trunk stabilized to help prevent injury. These types of muscles include interspinales, longissimus cervicis, iliocostalis thoracis, quadratus lumborum, and intertransversarii muscles.

11. C: The rotator cuff refers to the shoulder area. It is a large group of muscles and tendons that attach the humerus to the scapula. The tendons and muscles surround the humerus forming a cuff. The rotator cuff muscles are the supraspinatus, infraspinatus, teres minor, and subscapularis. These muscles are typically identified by the acronym SITS. The origin of these muscles is the scapula and the insertion is the humerus. These muscles all work synergistically but they also have unique functions. The supraspinatus muscle helps with abduction of the arm. The teres minor and the infraspinatus muscles help with the outward rotation of the arm. The subscapularis muscle helps with the medial rotation of the arm.

12. B: The atlantoaxial joint is a synovial joint (freely movable) that is subclassified as a pivot joint. This joint is located in the upper cervical area and allows for rotation of the head. The atlanto-occipital joint is a synovial gliding joint. This joint allows for nodding of the head. The costovertebral joint is also a synovial joint but is a gliding joint. This joint connects the ribs with the thoracic vertebrae. The intervertebral joint is a cartilaginous joint that is a gliding type joint. This allows for some limited movement between the vertebrae.

13. A: The medulla oblongata is the lowest part of the brainstem and is attached to the spinal cord. The medulla is considered to be the hindbrain along with the pons and cerebellum. The reticular formation is located within the medulla as are the olive and the pyramids. The medulla is also made up of white matter and gray matter. The pons connects the medulla to the midbrain. The medulla controls autonomic functions such as heart rate and breathing and also nonvital processes such as sneezing or vomiting. Any damage to the medulla oblongata is usually fatal.

14. A: The subdural space is located between the dura mater and the arachnoid mater. It contains only a small amount of cerebrospinal fluid (CSF) under normal conditions. If CSF is found within the subdural space, it is usually indicative of a pathological condition. The epidural space, subarachnoid space, spinal cord, and the ventricles of the brain all contain CSF. One purpose of CSF is to provide protection to the brain and spinal cord. It also provides a route of circulation for nutrients and helps to remove toxins or waste from the blood. CSF can also provide diagnostic information for certain types of neurological diseases.

15. D: Cranial nerves are numbered based on the order of connection to the brain, anterior to posterior. There are 12 pairs of cranial nerves: I. Olfactory; II. Optic; III. Oculomotor; IV. Trochlear; V. Trigeminal; VI. Abducens; VII. Facial; VIII. Vestibulocochlear; IX. Glossopharyngeal; X. Vagus; XI. Accessory; XII. Hypoglossal. Cranial nerves are comprised of axons with sensory, motor, or mixed functions. For example, the oculomotor nerve has motor function that regulates eye movements. The olfactory has sensory function for the sense of smell, and the glossopharyngeal has mixed functions for swallowing, sensations on the tongue, and reflex control of bodily processes such as blood pressure or respiration. There are mnemonic phrases available to help with the memorization of the names and functions of the 12 cranial nerves.

16. B: A plexus refers to a group of nerves intertwined together to form a network. Each plexus provides nerve impulses to specific areas of the body. The phrenic nerve is responsible for the contraction and relaxation of the diaphragm muscle. This nerve is located within the cervical plexus located in the neck. The brachial plexus is located in the shoulder region and supplies the nerve impulses to the lower shoulder and arms. The lumbar plexus is located in the lower back and the sacral plexus is located on the anterior surface of the pelvis. These two plexuses overlap and supply nerve impulses to the lower body including the thighs and legs.

17. D: The organs that are involved in the sense of balance are located in the inner ear: the vestibule and the semicircular canal. The crista ampullaris is located within the ampulla of the semicircular canal. Proper functioning of the crista ampullaris is required in order for normal dynamic equilibrium. Dynamic equilibrium refers to the ability to maintain balance when the head or body rotates quickly. The other type of equilibrium is static equilibrium. This refers to the ability to figure out the direction of the head related to gravity based on sense. Parts of the inner ear involved in static equilibrium are the macula, otoliths, and vestibular nerve fibers.

18. C: The sympathetic division of the autonomic nervous system is considered the emergency response of the human body commonly called "fight or flight." When in any kind of danger, the sympathetic division sends out signals to increase the physiologic response to stress. Examples of this would be an increase in heart rate and an increase in contraction of the heart in order to increase blood supply and oxygen to skeletal muscles. There would also be dilation of both the cardiac and skeletal blood vessels in order to receive the additional blood supply. Blood supply to the digestive system and spleen would be reduced and the blood vessels in this area would be constricted. Respiratory rate would increase. Glycogenolysis and lipolysis would also increase as a way to increase available glucose and fatty acids necessary for muscle cells.

19. A: The action of lifting a weight during a bicep curl is an example of a concentric contraction of a muscle. This occurs when the movement results in the shortening of a muscle fiber. The lowering of the weight during a bicep curl would be an eccentric contraction where the muscle fiber is lengthened during the movement. An isotonic contraction is when the tension remains the same but the length of the fiber changes, such as in the action of pushups. An isometric contraction is when the muscle length is same but the tension increases. A plank hold or other exercise where the position is held steady is an example of an isometric contraction.

20. C: Cardiac output is the volume of blood that leaves the ventricle in a given unit of time, such as mL per minute. Resting cardiac output is typically around 5000 mL/minute. This volume consists of approximately 700 mL/minute to the brain, 1000 mL/minute to the kidneys, 1250 mL/minute to the digestive tract, 1450 mL/minute to the skeletal muscles, 375 mL/minute to the skin, and 225 mL/minute into circulation. The level of cardiac output is directly influenced by the stroke volume (amount of blood pumped per heart beat) and the heart rate. Exercise works to improve cardiac output by making the heart beat stronger and faster. Conversely, many diseases or persistent activity will make the heart weaker and beat slower, thus reducing cardiac output.

21. B: Apnea is an interference or temporary disruption in breathing after a normal expiration. This condition may occur during sleeping, especially in severely overweight or obese individuals. Dyspnea is difficulty breathing, often as a result of increased carbon dioxide levels in the blood (hypoventilation). Hyperpnea is an increase in the level of breathing in order to improve oxygenation. This is also called hyperventilation. The term eupnea describes a normal breathing pattern with typical respiratory rate of approximately 12 to 17 breaths per minute. Cheyne-Stokes respiration is the type of labored, abnormal breathing seen most often in an individual who is close to death.

22. D: Urine formation occurs in the nephron. Urine is comprised of water, electrolytes, nitrogenous waste, toxins, and other components. The first step in the formation of urine is filtration. This occurs due to a pressure gradient from the glomeruli into the Bowman's capsule. Water and other solutes such as urea, chloride, and glucose are removed from the plasma in order to be filtered. The next step is reabsorption, which occurs in the proximal convoluted tubules. The majority of the water and other solutes that have been through the filtration process are moved back into circulation. A small volume is then left to enter the loop of Henle. Next reabsorption occurs in the loop of Henle, then in the distal tubules and collecting ducts. The final step in urine formation is tubular secretion when urea is secreted by diffusion in the loop of Henle. Ions such as hydrogen, potassium, and ammonium are also secreted by the distal tubules.

23. B: The liver is one of the most important organs in the human body. A person can live with a liver that is functioning at 10% of capacity; however, survival is not possible without any liver function. The liver is extremely important in many metabolic processes including the conversion of galactose and fructose into glucose. It also plays a major role in glycogenesis and glycogenolysis. Transamination and deamination of amino acids also occurs in the liver as well as synthesis of nonessential amino acids. Fatty acid oxidation occurs in the liver. The liver also produces many proteins, blood clotting factors, and enzymes as well as helping with the conversion of many vitamins. It provides storage for many vitamins including fat-soluble vitamins (A, D, E, K) and minerals, and it also produces and secretes bile. Bile is stored in the gall bladder. The liver metabolizes various steroids and provides detoxification for many drugs and toxins. The liver acts as a filter by removing various waste products and bacteria.

24. C: Growth hormone is produced by the pituitary gland. The direct action of growth hormone (also known as somatotropin) is to stimulate growth. This is done directly by promoting protein anabolism, which in turn leads to growth and development of new cells, muscles, bones, and many other types of tissues. Growth hormone (GH) also directly affects fat metabolism by stimulating the release of lipids from the adipose tissue. GH indirectly causes a rise in blood glucose levels because it causes the body to use lipids as the primary source of energy rather than glucose. A deficiency of GH during childhood can lead to short stature.

25. A: Glycolysis is an anaerobic pathway that occurs within cells. This process converts glucose into adenosine triphosphate (for energy) and pyruvic acid. This pathway does not require oxygen. Pyruvic acid is then converted into lactic acid as a byproduct of glycolysis. This step enables additional ATP to be produced. Glycolysis produces enough energy to fuel only a few seconds to a couple of minutes of high intensity exercise such as sprinting. When lactic acid builds up in the muscles, the lactate threshold is reached and muscle pain and burning result. Glycolysis is considered an inefficient energy pathway.

26. D: Gluconeogenesis is the formation of glucose from fatty acids or amino acids. In this process, pyruvate is converted into glucose. This process occurs mainly in the liver but also occurs to a lesser degree in the kidneys and small intestines. The process of gluconeogenesis is stimulated by cortisol, thyroxine, and other glucocorticoids. Since the glucose is made in the liver during this process, the liver releases this glucose into the blood stream as needed such as during sleep or periods of starvation. It is an important pathway because the brain requires a large amount of glucose every day.

27. B: Fatty acids that cannot be made in the human body are called essential fatty acids. These fatty acids must be obtained through food sources. The two essential fatty acids are linoleic and alpha-linolenic acid. Linoleic acid is from the omega-6 family and helps to reduce inflammation and is thought to be protective against heart disease. Alpha-linolenic acid is from the omega-3 family and is also protective against heart disease. Once consumed, these fatty acids can be converted into other polyunsaturated fatty acids such as eicosapentaenoic acid, docosahexaenoic acid and arachidonic acid. Good food sources of linoleic acid are vegetable oils such as corn, safflower, or sunflower oil. Food sources of alpha-linolenic acid are fatty fish, flaxseed, canola oil, and hemp seeds.

28. C: The process of protein digestion begins in the stomach after the food enters the mouth for chewing. The stomach secretes hydrochloric acid and pepsinogen, which interact to produce the enzyme pepsin. Pepsin is essential to protein digestion. Proteins are split into smaller units called polypeptides that are further split into amino acids. The majority of protein digestion takes place in the duodenum. The pancreas releases the enzyme trypsin, which works to break apart the amino acid bonds for absorption into circulation. Amino acids are then used for various functions such as growth and cell repair. There are 11 nonessential amino acids that can be produced within the body and 8 essential amino acids that must be consumed through the diet. The essential amino acids are histidine, isoleucine, leucine, lysine, methionine, phenylalanine, threonine, tryptophan and valine. Good protein sources are meat, fish, chicken, dairy, legumes, and beans.

29. D: The hormone glucagon is produced by the pancreas. It is secreted in response to hypoglycemia or very low blood sugar. It acts to raise glucose levels by stimulating the liver to convert glycogen into glucose. Glucagon also works to activate gluconeogenesis in the liver in order to provide another source of glucose in the body. Glucagon also has a role in breaking down triglycerides in the body into fatty acids that can also be used as fuel. Symptoms of hypoglycemia include blurred vision, confusion, shakiness, sweating, extreme hunger, and heart palpitations. Insulin has the opposite effect. It works to lower blood glucose levels in the body.

30. A: Vitamin D is needed by the body for calcium absorption and bone growth. It also plays a role in immune function, nervous system, and muscle contractions. Vitamin D can be obtained from fortified dairy products, some types of fish, egg yolks, and the sun. The risk for vitamin D deficiency can occur when the exposure to sunlight is reduced for a reason such as living in a northern climate or being homebound. Darker-skinned individuals also are at risk. Not consuming enough vitamin D–fortified food can lead to deficiency. Individuals with impaired kidney function may not be able to convert vitamin D to the active form needed in the body. Classic symptoms of vitamin D deficiency are rickets and osteomalacia, which may present as bone pain and muscle weakness. Symptoms may also include generalized aches and pains or feeling tired and lethargic; some individuals may not have any symptoms at all.

31. B: Potassium has many functions in the body including muscle contraction, acid-base balance, and controlling of electrical impulses of the heart. Potassium helps with blood pressure regulation. It also helps with growth, building of protein, and muscles. It is not considered an antioxidant. Examples of antioxidants are vitamin C, vitamin A, vitamin E, selenium, and beta-carotene. Potassium cannot be synthesized within the body and must be consumed in the diet. Good food sources of potassium include potatoes, broccoli, spinach, cantaloupe, bananas, oranges, and dairy products. Individuals who use certain diuretics, laxatives, or have severe vomiting or diarrhea may develop hypokalemia. Conversely, individuals with decreased kidney function or who take potassium-sparing diuretics may develop hyperkalemia.

32. C: The basal metabolic rate (BMR) is the amount of energy that is used while the body is considered at rest. The basal metabolic rate is measured when the body is in a resting state, at least 12 hours after the last meal, and at a comfortable temperature. There are many factors that affect the BMR. Males tend to have a higher BMR than females. People who are larger have higher BMRs than smaller people. Fever will raise the BMR. The thyroid hormones T_3 and T_4 affect BMR. Individuals with untreated hyperthyroid will have a higher BMR, and conversely, those with hypothyroid will have a lower BMR. The BMR also decreases with age. Certain types of drugs such as amphetamines or caffeine will increase the BMR.

33. B: Type 1 diabetes is considered an autoimmune disease in which the body's immune system mistakenly attacks its own beta cells on the pancreas, which are then rendered useless in their role of producing insulin. Cancer, Alzheimer disease, and Duchenne muscular dystrophy would all be considered diseases that are more cellular in nature. A cellular disease is one that occurs when some abnormal cells interfere with the normal functioning of the body. Cancer is one example, as evidenced by tumor growth of abnormal cells. Duchenne muscular dystrophy is an inherited disorder but is also a cellular disease. There is an abnormality within muscle cells where calcium enters the cells in an abnormal way, causing destruction of muscles. Alzheimer disease affects the neurons in the brain.

34. A: C-Reactive Protein (CRP) is a test used by physicians to measure general inflammation. High levels of CRP can indicate a flare-up of a preexisting inflammatory condition such as arthritis. A separate test, high-sensitivity C-reactive protein (hs-CRP) is a biochemical marker that is often used to evaluate vascular inflammation. It is typically measured in conjunction with other laboratory tests such as total cholesterol, LDL and HDL cholesterol, and triglycerides. An elevated hs-CRP has been correlated with an increased risk of cardiovascular disease including heart attack, sudden cardiac death, or stroke. Individuals who have a level towards the higher end of the normal range may have up to four times the risk for developing cardiac disease.

35. A: An autosomal recessive genetic condition is one where one copy of the defective gene must be passed along by each parent to the fetus in order for a condition to occur. If only one gene is passed along, the fetus would be a carrier of the condition. Cystic fibrosis is an example of an autosomal recessive gene. Other diseases are considered sex-linked, either dominant or recessive. A sex-linked dominant gene is one where the abnormal gene is passed along through either the X or Y chromosome and the fetus will definitely have the condition. This type is very rare. A sex-linked recessive gene such as the one that causes Duchenne muscular dystrophy must have two genes passed along for the condition to be present and usually refers to the Y chromosome. A single gene inheritance such as Huntington disease or Parkinson disease is controlled by one single gene.

36. D: The job of a normally functioning immune system is to protect the body from disease. In certain individuals, the immune system will actually attack the normal cells in the body, causing disease. Autoimmune diseases tend to be hereditary, and there is no known reason why this occurs. More than 80 autoimmune diseases are present, and obtaining an initial diagnosis can be a long and painful process because many of the symptoms are similar. General symptoms include feeling tired, running a low-grade fever, and muscle aches. The signs of an autoimmune disease that are considered "classic" are inflammation causing pain and swelling. Autoimmune diseases tend to have periods where there are flare-ups and remission. Examples of autoimmune disorders are multiple sclerosis, systemic lupus erythematosus (SLE), rheumatoid arthritis, and Grave's disease.

37. B: Osteoporosis is a disease where bones become brittle and weakened, potentially causing fractures. Caucasian and Asian women are at highest risk for developing osteoporosis but it can occur in anyone. Peak bone mass is achieved by most individuals in their early 20s. As individuals age, bone loss occurs. If peak bone mass was not optimal, chances for osteoporosis to occur increase. Other risk factors include family history, post menopausal state, poor calcium intake, altered eating habits such as anorexia nervosa, and weight-loss surgery. The use of steroid medication also increases the risk. Individuals who smoke, drink excessive alcohol, and have minimal exercise also increase their risk for developing the disease. Treatment typically involves calcium and vitamin D supplementation and bisphosphonate medications such as Fosamax to stimulate bone development. Treatment also includes weight-bearing exercises to help strengthen bones and prevention of falls to prevent fractures from occurring. Lifestyle changes such as smoking cessation and refraining from alcohol use are also encouraged.

38. D: A stroke or cerebrovascular accident (CVA) occurs when blood supply to the brain is disrupted causing brain cells to begin to die within minutes. A stroke may be caused by blocked arteries or a blood clot that makes its way to the brain. Individuals with hypertension, obesity, lack of exercise, heart disease, diabetes, smoking, and excessive alcohol use are at risk for a stroke to occur. Symptoms of a stroke include trouble with coordination, sudden confusion or difficulty speaking, paralysis, vision impairment, or a sudden, severe headache. A stroke that occurs on the right side of the brain will impact the left side of the body. Left-sided paralysis may occur along with vision impairment and memory loss. A stroke that occurs on the left side of the brain may cause right-sided paralysis, memory loss, speech impairment, and dysphagia (swallowing difficulty). It is imperative to act quickly if a stroke is in progress as early medical intervention can significantly improve outcome.

39. B: Synovial joints are the movable joints, also called diarthroses. These joints are further classified as uniaxial, biaxial, or multiaxial. The uniaxial joints include the knees or cervical vertebrae that allow the head to move. Biaxial joints include the thumb or finger joints. Multiaxial joints include the hip joint. Arthritis affects these types of joints. Arthritis can be caused by infections (bacterial or viral), severe physical stress, metabolic issues, or injury to the joint causing pain and inflammation. Osteoarthritis is typically a degenerative disease whereas rheumatoid arthritis is an inflammatory autoimmune disease. Symptoms include pain and stiffness of the affected joint causing limited range of motion. Certain pain-relieving medications such as analgesics or NSAIDs can be used to treat arthritis as well as exercises that improve range of motion and strengthen the muscles around the affected joints. In some cases, joint replacement surgery is required.

40. A: Microvascular complications such as nephropathy, neuropathy, and retinopathy are potential complications of poorly controlled diabetes mellitus. Nephropathy can begin to occur when albumin continues to spill into the urine causing microvascular damage in the kidneys. Untreated nephropathy can lead to severe kidney disease and the need for dialysis treatments. Retinopathy occurs when hyperglycemia damages the tiny vessels within the retina resulting in a reduction of oxygen flow to the retina. This causes a loss of vision over time. Neuropathy occurs when chronic hyperglycemia causes nerve damage to peripheral vessels. This can result in a lack of sensation in various parts of the body such as hands or feet. Neuropathy can also affect the gastrointestinal tract causing delayed gastric emptying or gastroparesis.

41. C: Blood pressure is measured as a reading of systolic pressure (when the heart is beating) and diastolic pressure (when the heart is at rest). Hypertension does not always present with definitive symptoms. Risk factors for hypertension include increasing age, African American heritage, obesity or excessive weight, and lack of physical activity. Cigarette smoking or other tobacco use as well as excessive alcohol use increases the risk for high blood pressure. Stress and certain medical conditions such as diabetes or kidney disease can also increase the risk. Normal blood pressure is considered to be below 120/80 mm Hg. Prehypertension is a systolic pressure of 120–139 mm Hg or a diastolic pressure of 80–89 mm Hg. Stage 1 hypertension is a systolic pressure of 140–159 mm Hg or a diastolic pressure of 90–99 mm Hg. Stage 2 hypertension is systolic pressure 160 mm Hg or above and a diastolic pressure of 100 mm Hg or above. A hypertensive crisis is a systolic pressure 180 mm Hg or above or a diastolic pressure 110 mm Hg or above. This requires immediate medical attention.

42. C: The immune system has many different types of cells and proteins within it and each has a specific job. A cytokine is a type of protein that is released by cells within the immune system to act on other cells or antigens by stimulating or interfering with their function. They are considered to be like messengers because they help parts of the immune system communicate with each other. Typically once cytokines are released an inflammation will follow. This is considered cell-mediated immunity. Examples of cytokines are interferon, leukotrienes, interleukin, tumor necrosis factor (TNF), and granulocyte colony-stimulating factor (G-CSF). The functions of cytokines are being studied closely by the pharmaceutical companies in order to produce biotechnology to help fight autoimmune diseases. For example, when leukotrienes are released after coming in contact with an allergen, the airway muscles become tight and excess mucus is then produced. Leukotriene modifiers are used to treat individuals with asthma by blocking the action of leukotrienes.

43. B: T cells and B cells are lymphocytes. Each has a specific job. T cells can be helper cells by sending chemical signals in the form of cytokines to help the other immune cells respond to a threat. T cells are part of the cell-mediated response. T cells can also be killer cells in that they attach themselves to the dangerous cells and release certain chemicals to destroy the pathogens inside the dangerous cells. B cells are the cells that produce and secrete the antibodies. Antibodies are specific proteins and will only bind to one specific type of antigen or protein. Specific antibodies work to find the specific antigens they are meant to attack. As antibodies are produced, a signal is sent to other cells to attack the foreign substance. B cells are part of humoral or antibody response.

44. D: There are many ways bacterial infections can be transmitted. One way is through a tick bite (called rickettsial). Rocky Mountain spotted fever is one of the most common rickettsial diseases reported. Initial symptoms are a sudden fever, muscle pain, and headache. A rash will develop soon after. Other methods of bacterially transmitted diseases include airborne transmission such as with tuberculosis. Another method is through eating contaminated food (fecal-oral route) such as with Salmonella, E. coli, Clostridioides difficile, cholera, or Campylobacter. Transmission can also be through sexual contact such as certain sexually transmitted diseases like syphilis or gonorrhea. Direct transmission through skin to skin contact is also a possibility such as with impetigo (group A streptococcus) or MRSA (methicillin-resistant Staphylococcus aureus).

45. A: The fecal-oral route of transmission refers to the spread of various forms of microbes such as bacteria, viruses, or parasites from the stool into the oral cavity. It is a very common mode of transmission for many diseases. Transmission occurs when an infected individual touches other items with contaminated hands, such as shaking someone else's hands or touching hard surfaces such as in the bathroom. The infected individual can also transmit through touching food such as raw vegetables or fruit. Transmission can also occur in the drinking water. Hepatitis A is transmitted this way. An infected individual can transmit hepatitis A even if no symptoms are present. Hepatitis A can infect the liver and cause inflammation. Hepatitis B is transmitted through a skin puncture or through contaminated bodily fluids. Hepatitis C is transmitted through contact with infected blood. Hepatitis D is also transmitted through a skin puncture or contamination with infected blood but can only be contracted by someone who already is infected with hepatitis B.

46. C: Giardiasis is caused by a parasitic infection called Giardia intestinalis. This parasite can be found in food, soil, or water. Swallowing contaminated water can cause significant gastrointestinal symptoms such as diarrhea lasting one to two weeks, abdominal pain and bloating, nausea, and flatulence. Giardia is now considered the most common cause of waterborne illness in the United States. Ingesting even a sip of water from a contaminated lake, stream, fountain, or hot tub can cause illness. Giardia can also survive for as long as 45 minutes in a chlorinated pool. It can also be transmitted from touching a surface that is contaminated with Giardia.

47. A: A dermatophyte is a fungus that causes infections affecting the skin, hair, or nails. One of these is commonly known as ringworm. Dermatophytes can thrive in wet or damp conditions such as on the skin, on different types of surfaces, and on many household items such as towels or sheets. Transmission is through direct contact. This is a very common infection and individuals can be healthy or have a weakened immune system. A symptom of a dermatophyte infection is an itchy area such as the legs, arms, scalp, groin, or nails. The area can appear red, cracked, or scaly. Infected nails can become thick and discolored and may disintegrate. An antifungal medication is required to treat the infection and may be needed for up to six weeks.

48. C: Group A streptococcus (GAS) is a type of bacteria that can be found in the throat or on the skin. Some individuals may be carriers of GAS but have no signs or symptoms of illness. Others may present with mild symptoms such as strep throat or impetigo, which is a type of skin infection. GAS can also progress to more severe symptoms such as necrotizing fasciitis or toxic shock syndrome. The majority of individuals who come in contact with GAS will only have mild symptoms, but individuals with chronic diseases or weakened immune systems may develop more serious symptoms. Early signs may be fever, confusion, flu-like symptoms, and dizziness. GAS requires treatment with antibiotics, and the more serious cases may require hospitalization. Good hand washing and good hygiene help prevent the spread of GAS. Any open wounds should be kept clean and closely monitored for signs of infection.

49. B: The Centers for Disease Control and Prevention (CDC) is a part of the United States Department of Health and Human Services. It has been in existence since 1946, and its primary goal is the preservation of public health with the use of monitoring, prevention, investigation into health issues when needed, education, promotion of healthy behaviors, and research. The CDC also provides training and leadership for many different areas and types of professions. The CDC demands accountability from all aspects that may affect overall public health, from outbreaks of food poisoning to a cluster of a certain type of cancer in a generalized location. There is a list of diseases that must be reported to the CDC that includes hepatitis, different strains of influenza, HIV/AIDS, sexually transmitted diseases, botulism, different types of food poisoning, and Lyme disease to name a few. The CDC is also on the front line for emergency preparedness and response to any emergency such as natural disasters or terrorism.

50. A: Infectious diseases can be very dangerous for certain people such as the elderly, the very young, or individuals with compromised immune systems. There are many infectious diseases that are considered emerging, such as SARS or West Nile virus, and others that are considered reemerging. Reemerging diseases are diseases that have previously been under control through prevention, vaccination, or drug treatment or are just generally persistent infectious diseases that have not been curtailed. Now diseases are returning that are resistant to drug therapy. Examples of reemerging diseases are mumps and infections of Streptococcus A, Staphylococcus aureus, enterovirus 71, and Clostridioides difficile.

How to Overcome Test Anxiety

Just the thought of taking a test is enough to make most people a little nervous. A test is an important event that can have a long-term impact on your future, so it's important to take it seriously and it's natural to feel anxious about performing well. But just because anxiety is normal, that doesn't mean that it's helpful in test taking, or that you should simply accept it as part of your life. Anxiety can have a variety of effects. These effects can be mild, like making you feel slightly nervous, or severe, like blocking your ability to focus or remember even a simple detail.

If you experience test anxiety—whether severe or mild—it's important to know how to beat it. To discover this, first you need to understand what causes test anxiety.

Causes of Test Anxiety

While we often think of anxiety as an uncontrollable emotional state, it can actually be caused by simple, practical things. One of the most common causes of test anxiety is that a person does not feel adequately prepared for their test. This feeling can be the result of many different issues such as poor study habits or lack of organization, but the most common culprit is time management. Starting to study too late, failing to organize your study time to cover all of the material, or being distracted while you study will mean that you're not well prepared for the test. This may lead to cramming the night before, which will cause you to be physically and mentally exhausted for the test. Poor time management also contributes to feelings of stress, fear, and hopelessness as you realize you are not well prepared but don't know what to do about it.

Other times, test anxiety is not related to your preparation for the test but comes from unresolved fear. This may be a past failure on a test, or poor performance on tests in general. It may come from comparing yourself to others who seem to be performing better or from the stress of living up to expectations. Anxiety may be driven by fears of the future—how failure on this test would affect your educational and career goals. These fears are often completely irrational, but they can still negatively impact your test performance.

Elements of Test Anxiety

As mentioned earlier, test anxiety is considered to be an emotional state, but it has physical and mental components as well. Sometimes you may not even realize that you are suffering from test anxiety until you notice the physical symptoms. These can include trembling hands, rapid heartbeat, sweating, nausea, and tense muscles. Extreme anxiety may lead to fainting or vomiting. Obviously, any of these symptoms can have a negative impact on testing. It is important to recognize them as soon as they begin to occur so that you can address the problem before it damages your performance.

The mental components of test anxiety include trouble focusing and inability to remember learned information. During a test, your mind is on high alert, which can help you recall information and stay focused for an extended period of time. However, anxiety interferes with your mind's natural processes, causing you to blank out, even on the questions you know well. The strain of testing during anxiety makes it difficult to stay focused, especially on a test that may take several hours. Extreme anxiety can take a huge mental toll, making it difficult not only to recall test information but even to understand the test questions or pull your thoughts together.

Effects of Test Anxiety

Test anxiety is like a disease—if left untreated, it will get progressively worse. Anxiety leads to poor performance, and this reinforces the feelings of fear and failure, which in turn lead to poor performances on subsequent tests. It can grow from a mild nervousness to a crippling condition. If allowed to progress, test anxiety can have a big impact on your schooling, and consequently on your future.

Test anxiety can spread to other parts of your life. Anxiety on tests can become anxiety in any stressful situation, and blanking on a test can turn into panicking in a job situation. But fortunately, you don't have to let anxiety rule your testing and determine your grades. There are a number of relatively simple steps you can take to move past anxiety and function normally on a test and in the rest of life.

Physical Steps for Beating Test Anxiety

While test anxiety is a serious problem, the good news is that it can be overcome. It doesn't have to control your ability to think and remember information. While it may take time, you can begin taking steps today to beat anxiety.

Just as your first hint that you may be struggling with anxiety comes from the physical symptoms, the first step to treating it is also physical. Rest is crucial for having a clear, strong mind. If you are tired, it is much easier to give in to anxiety. But if you establish good sleep habits, your body and mind will be ready to perform optimally, without the strain of exhaustion. Additionally, sleeping well helps you to retain information better, so you're more likely to recall the answers when you see the test questions.

Getting good sleep means more than going to bed on time. It's important to allow your brain time to relax. Take study breaks from time to time so it doesn't get overworked, and don't study right before bed. Take time to rest your mind before trying to rest your body, or you may find it difficult to fall asleep.

Along with sleep, other aspects of physical health are important in preparing for a test. Good nutrition is vital for good brain function. Sugary foods and drinks may give a burst of energy but this burst is followed by a crash, both physically and emotionally. Instead, fuel your body with protein and vitamin-rich foods.

Also, drink plenty of water. Dehydration can lead to headaches and exhaustion, especially if your brain is already under stress from the rigors of the test. Particularly if your test is a long one, drink water during the breaks. And if possible, take an energy-boosting snack to eat between sections.

Along with sleep and diet, a third important part of physical health is exercise. Maintaining a steady workout schedule is helpful, but even taking 5-minute study breaks to walk can help get your blood pumping faster and clear your head. Exercise also releases endorphins, which contribute to a positive feeling and can help combat test anxiety.

When you nurture your physical health, you are also contributing to your mental health. If your body is healthy, your mind is much more likely to be healthy as well. So take time to rest, nourish your body with healthy food and water, and get moving as much as possible. Taking these physical steps will make you stronger and more able to take the mental steps necessary to overcome test anxiety.

Mental Steps for Beating Test Anxiety

Working on the mental side of test anxiety can be more challenging, but as with the physical side, there are clear steps you can take to overcome it. As mentioned earlier, test anxiety often stems from lack of preparation, so the obvious solution is to prepare for the test. Effective studying may be the most important weapon you have for beating test anxiety, but you can and should employ several other mental tools to combat fear.

First, boost your confidence by reminding yourself of past success—tests or projects that you aced. If you're putting as much effort into preparing for this test as you did for those, there's no reason you should expect to fail here. Work hard to prepare; then trust your preparation.

Second, surround yourself with encouraging people. It can be helpful to find a study group, but be sure that the people you're around will encourage a positive attitude. If you spend time with others who are anxious or cynical, this will only contribute to your own anxiety. Look for others who are motivated to study hard from a desire to succeed, not from a fear of failure.

Third, reward yourself. A test is physically and mentally tiring, even without anxiety, and it can be helpful to have something to look forward to. Plan an activity following the test, regardless of the outcome, such as going to a movie or getting ice cream.

When you are taking the test, if you find yourself beginning to feel anxious, remind yourself that you know the material. Visualize successfully completing the test. Then take a few deep, relaxing breaths and return to it. Work through the questions carefully but with confidence, knowing that you are capable of succeeding.

Developing a healthy mental approach to test taking will also aid in other areas of life. Test anxiety affects more than just the actual test—it can be damaging to your mental health and even contribute to depression. It's important to beat test anxiety before it becomes a problem for more than testing.

Study Strategy

Being prepared for the test is necessary to combat anxiety, but what does being prepared look like? You may study for hours on end and still not feel prepared. What you need is a strategy for test prep. The next few pages outline our recommended steps to help you plan out and conquer the challenge of preparation.

Step 1: Scope Out the Test

Learn everything you can about the format (multiple choice, essay, etc.) and what will be on the test. Gather any study materials, course outlines, or sample exams that may be available. Not only will this help you to prepare, but knowing what to expect can help to alleviate test anxiety.

Step 2: Map Out the Material

Look through the textbook or study guide and make note of how many chapters or sections it has. Then divide these over the time you have. For example, if a book has 15 chapters and you have five days to study, you need to cover three chapters each day. Even better, if you have the time, leave an extra day at the end for overall review after you have gone through the material in depth.

If time is limited, you may need to prioritize the material. Look through it and make note of which sections you think you already have a good grasp on, and which need review. While you are studying, skim quickly through the familiar sections and take more time on the challenging parts.

Write out your plan so you don't get lost as you go. Having a written plan also helps you feel more in control of the study, so anxiety is less likely to arise from feeling overwhelmed at the amount to cover.

Step 3: Gather Your Tools

Decide what study method works best for you. Do you prefer to highlight in the book as you study and then go back over the highlighted portions? Or do you type out notes of the important information? Or is it helpful to make flashcards that you can carry with you? Assemble the pens, index cards, highlighters, post-it notes, and any other materials you may need so you won't be distracted by getting up to find things while you study.

If you're having a hard time retaining the information or organizing your notes, experiment with different methods. For example, try color-coding by subject with colored pens, highlighters, or post-it notes. If you learn better by hearing, try recording yourself reading your notes so you can listen while in the car, working out, or simply sitting at your desk. Ask a friend to quiz you from your flashcards, or try teaching someone the material to solidify it in your mind.

Step 4: Create Your Environment

It's important to avoid distractions while you study. This includes both the obvious distractions like visitors and the subtle distractions like an uncomfortable chair (or a too-comfortable couch that makes you want to fall asleep). Set up the best study environment possible: good lighting and a comfortable work area. If background music helps you focus, you may want to turn it on, but otherwise keep the room quiet. If you are using a computer to take notes, be sure you don't have any other windows open, especially applications like social media, games, or anything else that could distract you. Silence your phone and turn off notifications. Be sure to keep water close by so you stay hydrated while you study (but avoid unhealthy drinks and snacks).

Also, take into account the best time of day to study. Are you freshest first thing in the morning? Try to set aside some time then to work through the material. Is your mind clearer in the afternoon or evening? Schedule your study session then. Another method is to study at the same time of day that you will take the test, so that your brain gets used to working on the material at that time and will be ready to focus at test time.

Step 5: Study!

Once you have done all the study preparation, it's time to settle into the actual studying. Sit down, take a few moments to settle your mind so you can focus, and begin to follow your study plan. Don't give in to distractions or let yourself procrastinate. This is your time to prepare so you'll be ready to fearlessly approach the test. Make the most of the time and stay focused.

Of course, you don't want to burn out. If you study too long you may find that you're not retaining the information very well. Take regular study breaks. For example, taking five minutes out of every hour to walk briskly, breathing deeply and swinging your arms, can help your mind stay fresh.

As you get to the end of each chapter or section, it's a good idea to do a quick review. Remind yourself of what you learned and work on any difficult parts. When you feel that you've mastered the material, move on to the next part. At the end of your study session, briefly skim through your notes again.

But while review is helpful, cramming last minute is NOT. If at all possible, work ahead so that you won't need to fit all your study into the last day. Cramming overloads your brain with more information than it can process and retain, and your tired mind may struggle to recall even previously learned information when it is overwhelmed with last-minute study. Also, the urgent nature of cramming and the stress placed on your brain contribute to anxiety. You'll be more likely to go to the test feeling unprepared and having trouble thinking clearly.

So don't cram, and don't stay up late before the test, even just to review your notes at a leisurely pace. Your brain needs rest more than it needs to go over the information again. In fact, plan to finish your studies by noon or early afternoon the day before the test. Give your brain the rest of the day to relax or focus on other things, and get a good night's sleep. Then you will be fresh for the test and better able to recall what you've studied.

Step 6: Take a Practice Test

Many courses offer sample tests, either online or in the study materials. This is an excellent resource to check whether you have mastered the material, as well as to prepare for the test format and environment.

Check the test format ahead of time: the number of questions, the type (multiple choice, free response, etc.), and the time limit. Then create a plan for working through them. For example, if you have 30 minutes to take a 60-question test, your limit is 30 seconds per question. Spend less time on the questions you know well so that you can take more time on the difficult ones.

If you have time to take several practice tests, take the first one open book, with no time limit. Work through the questions at your own pace and make sure you fully understand them. Gradually work up to taking a test under test conditions: sit at a desk with all study materials put away and set a timer. Pace yourself to make sure you finish the test with time to spare and go back to check your answers if you have time.

After each test, check your answers. On the questions you missed, be sure you understand why you missed them. Did you misread the question (tests can use tricky wording)? Did you forget the information? Or was it something you hadn't learned? Go back and study any shaky areas that the practice tests reveal.

Taking these tests not only helps with your grade, but also aids in combating test anxiety. If you're already used to the test conditions, you're less likely to worry about it, and working through tests until you're scoring well gives you a confidence boost. Go through the practice tests until you feel comfortable, and then you can go into the test knowing that you're ready for it.

Test Tips

On test day, you should be confident, knowing that you've prepared well and are ready to answer the questions. But aside from preparation, there are several test day strategies you can employ to maximize your performance.

First, as stated before, get a good night's sleep the night before the test (and for several nights before that, if possible). Go into the test with a fresh, alert mind rather than staying up late to study.

Try not to change too much about your normal routine on the day of the test. It's important to eat a nutritious breakfast, but if you normally don't eat breakfast at all, consider eating just a protein bar. If you're a coffee drinker, go ahead and have your normal coffee. Just make sure you time it so that the caffeine doesn't wear off right in the middle of your test. Avoid sugary beverages, and drink enough water to stay hydrated but not so much that you need a restroom break 10 minutes into the test. If your test isn't first thing in the morning, consider going for a walk or doing a light workout before the test to get your blood flowing.

Allow yourself enough time to get ready, and leave for the test with plenty of time to spare so you won't have the anxiety of scrambling to arrive in time. Another reason to be early is to select a good seat. It's helpful to sit away from doors and windows, which can be distracting. Find a good seat, get out your supplies, and settle your mind before the test begins.

When the test begins, start by going over the instructions carefully, even if you already know what to expect. Make sure you avoid any careless mistakes by following the directions.

Then begin working through the questions, pacing yourself as you've practiced. If you're not sure on an answer, don't spend too much time on it, and don't let it shake your confidence. Either skip it and come back later, or eliminate as many wrong answers as possible and guess among the remaining ones. Don't dwell on these questions as you continue—put them out of your mind and focus on what lies ahead.

Be sure to read all of the answer choices, even if you're sure the first one is the right answer. Sometimes you'll find a better one if you keep reading. But don't second-guess yourself if you do immediately know the answer. Your gut instinct is usually right. Don't let test anxiety rob you of the information you know.

If you have time at the end of the test (and if the test format allows), go back and review your answers. Be cautious about changing any, since your first instinct tends to be correct, but make sure you didn't misread any of the questions or accidentally mark the wrong answer choice. Look over any you skipped and make an educated guess.

At the end, leave the test feeling confident. You've done your best, so don't waste time worrying about your performance or wishing you could change anything. Instead, celebrate the successful completion of this test. And finally, use this test to learn how to deal with anxiety even better next time.

Review Video: Test Anxiety
Visit mometrix.com/academy and enter code: 100340

Important Qualification

Not all anxiety is created equal. If your test anxiety is causing major issues in your life beyond the classroom or testing center, or if you are experiencing troubling physical symptoms related to your anxiety, it may be a sign of a serious physiological or psychological condition. If this sounds like your situation, we strongly encourage you to seek professional help.

Online Resources

Due to our efforts to try to keep this book to a manageable length, we've created a link that will give you access to all of your online resources:

mometrix.com/resources719/nbceparti

It's Your Moment, Let's Celebrate It!

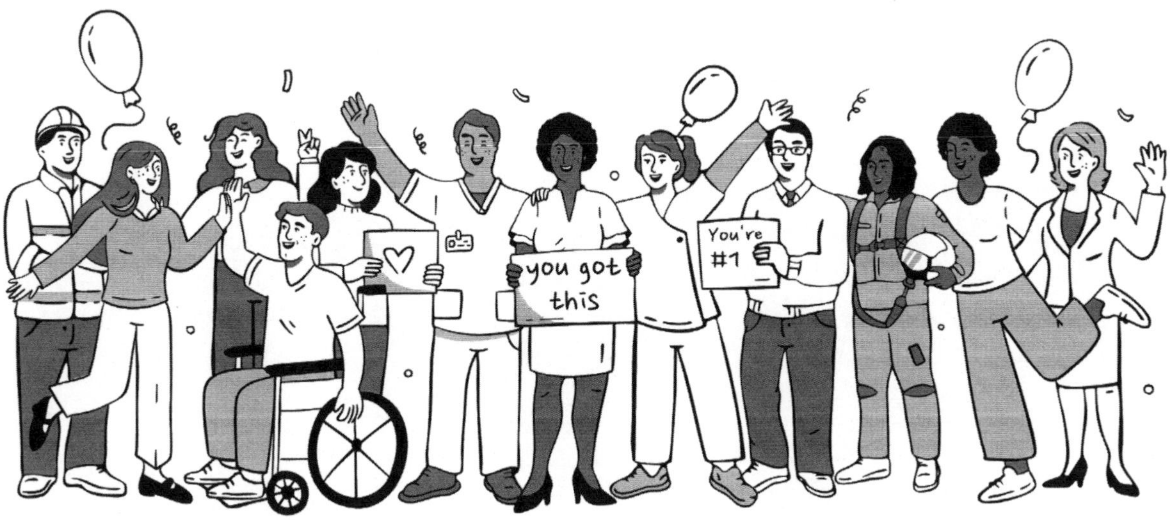

Share your story @mometrixtestpreparation